PREVENTING SENIOR MOMENTS

PREVENTING SENIOR MOMENTS

MOMENTS

How to Stay Alert into Your 90s and Beyond

STAN GOLDBERG

ROWMAN & LITTLEFIELD
Lanham • Boulder • New York • London

Published by Rowman & Littlefield
An imprint of The Rowman & Littlefield Publishing Group, Inc.
4501 Forbes Boulevard, Suite 200, Lanham, Maryland 20706
www.rowman.com
86-90 Paul Street, London EC2A 4NE
Copyright © 2023 by Stan Goldberg

British Library Cataloguing in Publication Information Available

Library of Congress Cataloging-in-Publication Data
ISBN: 978-1-5381-6941-4 (cloth)
ISBN: 978-1-5381-6942-1 (electronic)

Contents

Preface vii

Part I: The Basics 1
CHAPTER 1: Myths and Types of Senior Moments 3
CHAPTER 2: How Senior Moments Are Created 15
CHAPTER 3: A Very Short Primer on Memory 25
Part II: Strategies 33
CHAPTER 4: Slow Down 35
CHAPTER 5: Combating Inertia 53
CHAPTER 6: Patterns 65
CHAPTER 7: Challenge Your Brain 75
CHAPTER 8: Fortifying and Retrieving Memories 89
CHAPTER 9: Focus 97
CHAPTER 10: Managing Your Environment 107
CHAPTER 11: Practice, Practice, Practice 123
Part III: The Extras **135**
CHAPTER 12: Attitudes Needing Adjustment 137
CHAPTER 13: Sleep 149
CHAPTER 14: Feeding Your Brain 167
CHAPTER 15: When It Is More Serious Than a Senior
Moment 175

Contents

Chapter 16: Frequently Asked Questions 187

Chapter 17: Final Thoughts 193

Notes. 197

Bibliography 219

Index 243

About the Author 251

Preface

As a clinician in the area of communicative disorders and a counselor for seniors for thirty years, I tested the strategies and methods in this book with clients and myself. You will find endnotes throughout the book that cite the research on which my recommendations are based. Some strategies and methods that I hoped would become "magic bullets" were miserable failures. They do not appear in this book. Others, which I initially ignored because they were so simple, proved immensely successful. They do appear in the book. If you are interested in research, definitely look at the citations. If you are not, just ignore the numbers.

You will find many examples in each chapter. All are based either on my experiences, or the experiences of clients with whom I have worked. My clients' identities and names have been changed to protect their privacy.

Now, one further caveat—how I refer to the brain. I do not give brains endearing names, but I do attribute human characteristics to them, such as distractible, focused, intense, etc. I use these human qualities only to make the brain's information processing features more accessible to readers with little or no neurological background. So relax, my neuroscientist friends; I know the brain is neither friendly nor inquisitive.

PART I

THE BASICS

The way to get started is to quit talking and begin doing.
—WALT DISNEY

YOU ARE ABOUT TO GET INTIMATE WITH YOUR BRAIN. YOU KNOW a little about it since it has been around since you were born. On many occasions, you experienced delight when it created an unexpected, wonderful event, but maybe you pretended it was not yours when an outrageous senior moment resulted in an embarrassing story your friends still tell. You listened to experts explaining how neurons (or something else whose name you cannot pronounce) have more connections in the brain than there are grains of sand on all of Earth's beaches. You marveled how something weighing only three pounds can outperform the most powerful computer yet remain so versatile that, after solving a complex problem, it links a Burger King commercial to a forgotten experience that makes you cry.

You have many questions about this mysterious organ composed of 60 percent fat, such as why can you remember everything that occurred at a summer camp fifty years ago but not what you had for breakfast today. The journey you are about to take promises much—explanations of why you do what you do, how your brain works, and most importantly, how to eliminate senior moments. So buckle up, say hello to your brain, and in the words of Walt Disney, let's get started.

Myths and Types of Senior Moments

An amateur astronomer tells his senior friend the comet they are observing is more than six million miles away. The friend asks, "Is that from here or your house?"

Everyone has said or done something they immediately regretted, like forgetting the name of a granddaughter, misusing a common word, making a bizarre connection between events, or forgetting how to get to a favorite shopping mall. As we age, the number of these occurrences increases. We call them "senior moments," a phrase described in books and on social media as humorous statements or behaviors said or done by people over sixty.

Yes, some senior moments are laughable, like the question I asked my friend about the distance to the comet. Likewise, your senior moments may also have been the basis of jokes, qualified by soothing words such as, "Don't be upset; we're laughing *with* you, not *at* you." But other senior moments have consequences, like a grandson's expression of pain when his grandmother calls him by his brother's name or the distress a client experienced when she could not remember the route to her daughter's house. Most approaches to senior moments suggest we accept them as an inevitable, laughable part of aging. But what if you do not find humor in the humiliation, concern, or pain a senior moment causes you, your friends, or your family? What if you want to prevent them—then what? Agatha Christie's fictional detective Hercule Poirot would suggest starting by eliminating the "red herrings," or in the case of senior moments, the myths.

MYTHS

A student asked Roshi Jiyu-Kennett, the late Abbess of the Shasta Buddhist Monastery, how one can learn the meaning of life. The young novitiate patiently waited for a gem of knowledge that would change his life. After thinking for a while, Roshi said life was like a tasty glass of beer; you can enjoy the brew only after blowing off the useless suds.[1] The same millennium-old wisdom of eliminating what is not germane applies to senior moments.

So let us begin by debunking six foamy myths that, unfortunately, have lent credence to the popular belief that senior moments are an inevitable and unchangeable part of aging. Let's explore the following ideas:

1. Senior moments are momentary brain glitches confined to seniors.

2. All senior moments can be grouped together.

3. Senior moments are solely the result of memory problems.

4. Senior moments are an inevitable part of aging.

5. Senior moments should be no more concerning than a good laugh.

6. Senior moments are isolated events that do not define who you are.

Momentary Brain Glitches Confined to Seniors

The phrase "senior moment" implies that the event is confined to one age group and is short in duration. However, senior moments are neither limited to people over sixty nor fleeting. Yes, they occur more often in seniors. Still, there is no age starting line.[2] The word "moment" implies that senior moments are blips that pop up without connections to what precedes the event and vanish when it ends. But there are *always* precursors to senior moments. Think about one senior moment that stands out, like forgetting an important appointment. How well did you sleep the night before the appointment? Was there something pressing occupying your mind? Were you still reeling from a comment made about you by a colleague? If you search, you will find that at least one causative event preceded your senior moment. If you cannot find one, you have not looked hard enough.

All Senior Moments Can Be Grouped Together

Did you know there are nine types of senior moments? Probably not, since *Preventing Senior Moments* is the first book in which these distinctions appear. Until now, senior moments were thought to be so indistinguishable from each other that all could be lumped into a single category. After all, forgetting where you put your glasses for the umpteenth time is as embarrassing as conflating memories into something that never happened. Yes, *forgetting objects* and *conflating memories* are examples of senior moments, but lumping them together hides significant differences that will affect their prevention. It would be like trying to understand nutrition by labeling sugar, oranges, tomatoes, celery, and a fatty piece of steak just as "food." Yes, all are foods, but some will bolster your energy while others may make you a candidate for a quadruple bypass.

Senior Moments Are Solely the Result of Memory Problems

Memory loss plays a significant role in creating many, but not all, senior moments. To add some more complexity to our understanding of memory, the kind of memory loss found in many senior moments differs. It is not helpful to simply say, "She has memory issues," when someone conflates two events into one that never existed. It is more informative to determine if a memory issue caused the senior moment, and if it did, what type of problem was the culprit. For example, not remembering why I am in the kitchen after leaving my office (sequential memory) is different from not realizing I already told the same story (short-term memory) fifteen minutes ago.

Senior Moments Are an Inevitable Part of Aging

Not quite. Yes, senior moments tend to occur more often as we age, but they are not inevitable, and linking them to aging is not helpful. It would be like linking longevity to a healthy lifestyle without identifying the responsible components of that lifestyle. The inevitability conclusion is often based on how an older brain functions without compensatory strategies. We are all susceptible to the aging process. Muscles will shrink whether you are a professional bodybuilder or someone whose idea of bodybuilding is taking out the garbage once a week. While some seniors struggle with their senior moments as if trapped in a locked room, others have learned strategies to compensate for the changes. Strategies enable them to function as they did when much younger—as they will for you.

We cannot prevent aging, but we can coax the brain to process information at age seventy-five as it did when we were in our fifties *if we give it a little help*. It is similar to a new Tesla and a 1959 Edsel traveling to the same destination three hundred miles away. The Tesla driver will make the trip without stopping for gas or repairs. The Edsel driver will probably need to stop to repair a hose line, add water to the radiator, gas up, and determine why smoke is gushing out from under the hood. Both cars will make it to their destination in different ways, times, and days.

Senior Moments Should Be No More Concerning Than a Good Laugh

Losing one's glasses two or three times a day might be great fodder for a late-night comedian's opening monologue. But there is no humor when your senior moment makes others question your cognitive ability. It happened to me when I could not remember the title of my last book during a live broadcast interview.

I am sure you can recall a senior moment that was genuinely humorous. I have had too many to list, even if I could remember them. But other senior moments were more concerning, like not remembering my zip code when it was the precursor for using a credit card at a gas station. Despite having lived at the same address for more than forty years, I could only remember the first two numbers. The harder I tried, the more distant the last digits became. There was nothing humorous about my senior moment since I had little cash and other drivers were impatiently waiting for gas. Once you understand the genesis of a senior moment and what it may imply about your information processing skills, most will lose their hilarity.

Senior Moments Are Isolated Events That Do Not Define Who You Are

Our identity is an amalgam of behaviors, beliefs, history, and expectations. Psychologists such as Erik Erikson viewed it as a "gestalt," the wholeness of who you are.[3] Sociologists such as Henri Talfel believed that identity also includes how a person relates to others, which includes senior moments.[4] However, the most poignant view of identity was depicted in a 1930s cartoon. Popeye stands on the bow of a small boat in the middle of a storm, Sweet Pea rows and Bluto looks at a menu.[5] "I'm Popeye the Sailor Man," Popeye says. "And I yam what I yam, and that's what I yam." The words and actions of each cartoon character unequivocally signal to the audience their identity: Popeye, the leader who does little of importance other than telling people who he is; Bluto, whose gluttony overshadows the need to row during a storm; and Sweet Pea ignored by both men as she valiantly tries to save everyone.

Just as the cartoon characters' words and behaviors contribute to their identities, so do your senior moments participate in yours. As much as you would like to think senior moments are not a part of you, they are. It would be great if we could separate those parts of us that we do not like from those we cherish; our embarrassing senior moments from our brilliant ideas. Sadly, it is a package deal, a gumbo whose many ingredients combine to form a distinctive, one-of-a-kind flavor. Remove an ingredient, and the flavor changes. Add some filé and the character of the stew becomes different.

Now that you know what senior moments are not, you want to know what they are. First, there are nine types of senior moments. You probably have not considered your senior moments to be different, since they are embarrassing or concerning no matter how we classify them. That is true, but by understanding their uniqueness, you will learn how to select the most appropriate strategies and methods for preventing them. It is similar to cutting-edge approaches for fighting cancer, where the type of cancer determines the intervention protocol.

Types of Senior Moments

There are nine types of senior moments that, while distinct, are tied together by information processing errors. The complexity of the relationship is similar to a lesson taught to me by my father when I was a child in the 1950s. Every Friday I would help my father make sausage in the family grocery store. We gathered meats that had not been sold during the week and dumped them into a grinder. By changing some of the spices or the percentage of pork, beef, or lamb, what emerged was Italian hot sausage, kielbasa, Polish sausage, bratwurst, and something my father called "Irving's Special." Think of senior moments as similar to sausages. All senior moments have something in common—they arose because of an information processing error. Like my father's sausages, they differ in the specifics, like memory, physiology, experience, etc.

Clients have shared with me an amazing number of senior moments. Some were humorous, like telling a hilarious joke at a party and having nobody laugh—since he had also just told it twenty minutes before. But others were disturbing, like not remembering how to return home after driving to a new destination. The hundreds of senior moment stories I heard fell into the following nine categories.

Forgetting Names or Numbers

How often have you been at a party, and a person approaches you whose name has inexplicably been stripped from your memory? While you may be able to dance around not knowing their name if it was just the two of you, your partner is present, and an introduction will be necessary. As the nameless person approaches, your anxiety exponentially increases with each step. You race through the alphabet or try to make an association that will trigger their name. *Ok, their hair is cut short, maybe "Shorty?" or "Sherman" because that name begins with an S, and so does "short hair."* The machinations continue until they are right in front of you. You go from panic mode to survival, turn to your partner and say, "You know each other, right?" The consequence of forgetting a name in our example might be just embarrassment. But other events, like forgetting your spouse's birthday, may affect your relationship.

Repeating Stories and Asking Questions

You are at a party and someone begins telling a fascinating story about a trip to Alaska. You and most other people listening groan and prepare to hear the story for the second time that night and the fourth time this month. Is it dementia, you wonder? Possibly, but more likely the repetition of the story has more to do with the significance it has in the person's life coupled with a short-term memory problem than it does with Alzheimer's.

Misplacing Objects

We all misplace objects. It is a daily occurrence for some people, often involving the same object. For example, a client lost her glasses almost daily and spent a ridiculous amount of time trying to find them. Fortunately, the glasses always appeared in the usual places: at the bottom of her purse, on a kitchen table, in a drawer, or in a jacket pocket. Her husband knew the first words she would say after they drove less than a block would be, "Wait, I forgot my glasses!" He would smile, continue driving, and list each place her glasses "decided" to hide. Although everyone laughed when the husband told the story, his wife found nothing humorous about being treated like a five-year-old.

Substituting Words

When a man asked his wife if their dog, George, had been fed, he used a long-deceased pet's name, followed by the name of another dead dog, then a third, eventually retrieving "George." During conversations, people may substitute one word for another. The usual response is laughter, as it was with my client. However, the reaction would have been very different if, instead of asking if George had been fed, he asked if "New York" had been fed. The reason for concern would be that the substitution would have come from a different semantic class (name of a city). This type of substitution would have signaled a possible neurological problem.[6]

Sequencing Problems

Everyone has experienced problems with tasks that require a series of steps, such as moving a paragraph within a document. For me to do it on my computer, I need to follow six steps.

1. Identify the change I want to make.

2. Determine where I will move the paragraph.

3. Highlight the paragraph so the computer knows what to move.

4. Cut the paragraph.

5. Locate the insertion point where I want to place the paragraph.

6. Paste the entry.

Sometimes, if the sequence is interrupted for as little as thirty seconds, I forget the reason for initiating the move. For example, when my dog came to my side and licked my hand after I cut the paragraph, I forgot where I wanted to place the excerpt. The problem of correctly sequencing a task also occurs in other areas, such as forgetting why I was in the kitchen after leaving my office, why I made a turn while driving, or where I was in cooking a multistep entree.

Difficulty Completing Tasks

It is Saturday morning, and you look at a list of unfinished projects that have been accumulating for the last six months. The garage is so disorganized you cannot find any of the necessary tools. The garden, which at one time was your pride and joy, is overgrown with weeds that are sucking the life out of your daffodils. You look at piles of papers on your desk, and spot incomplete thank-you notes for a party you gave three months ago. You are so overwhelmed that instead of starting any of the tasks, you curl up in your favorite chair and begin reading a new novel.

Procrastination is often seen as a major reason seniors do not complete tasks.[7] However, what may appear to be procrastination might actually be your inability to multitask. You may have been adept at juggling three or more projects simultaneously when you were forty. However, at seventy, your ability to successfully attend to more than one task at a time has seriously deteriorated.

Conflating Memories

A person asked someone to describe a ten-year-old incident he did not witness. The speaker entertained the listener with a story that sounded believable. However, the story dumbfounded his partner because what he described was actually a mixture of three different events, a scenario as bizarre as the land depicted in *The Wizard of Oz*.

As we get older, there is an increased possibility of melding memories into an event that never occurred.[8] While some people would label these as deliberate lies, fabrications, or exaggerations, many of these result from our brain physiology rather than deliberate attempts to deceive. Physiologically, the brain is not programmed to retrieve a perfectly accurate rendition of something that happened in the past.[9] The creation of a nonexistent event may result from how the aging brain responds to a retrieval request.

Difficulty Understanding

A person in her sixties had problems understanding fast-talking customer service representatives with foreign accents. Comprehension became so arduous that she allowed all calls to go to voice mail and later repeatedly listened until she understood them. Friends and family would often joke when calling her. "Pick up the phone, Harriet. I'm not a telemarketer!" Various conditions can impair understanding, ranging from dead hearing aid batteries to a brain tumor. Most are not as minor as the first or as frightening as the second.

Disorientation

A contractor who shopped at Home Depot visited the hardware section so regularly over thirty years that he did not have to think about the location of screws. It seemed as if his legs were programmed to take him to Section 6, Aisle 4, Shelf 2. However, on one particular day, when shopping for screws, he drew a blank on their location.

Disorientation is a psychological condition that develops when the structure of your world begins to evaporate.[10] Structure is the set of rules—some obvious, others implied—that guide our personal interactions and make the world understandable. Some are scripted, such as a state agency's pamphlet on how to drive a car. Others are unwritten social norms, such as greeting rituals, that are passed down through generations. The disappearance or corruption of structure can be consequential. According to many people, disorientation is the most disturbing type of senior moment, not only because it is psychologically disruptive, but it suggests the onset of dementia.[11]

CHAPTER 2

How Senior Moments Are Created

All events and incidents in life are so intimately linked with the
fate of others that a single person on his or her own cannot
even begin to act.

—His Holiness, the Dalai Lama[1]

THE DALAI LAMA'S VIEW ON THE INTERCONNECTIVITY OF ALL
people lays the foundation for explaining why things happen
in general and specifically why you experience senior moments.
How often have you had a senior moment that was inexplicable
to you and to those who witnessed it? You thought, *how could*
that have happened? How could I have done something so ridiculous?
Your friends and family may have been less kind, thinking, *She's*
losing her mind! To understand why senior moments occur, we
need to adopt the millennium-old Buddhist concept of dependent
origination.

Dependent origination states if you want to understand an
event or person, you must look at its history. Nothing, according
to this belief, just "pops up." Western scientists latched on to this
doctrine, reframing it as the "principle of causation."[2] If you can
identify the cause of a senior moment, you are 80 percent on the
way to preventing it. You will find that every one of your senior

moments originated from **(1) an information processing hiccup or (2) one of two bad actors that are determined to embarrass you.**

INFORMATION PROCESSING HICCUPS

The brain processes information in five sequential steps: **(1) attending, (2) making sense, (3) storing, (4) retrieving, and (5) using**. A senior moment may occur if a problem exists in any of these steps. Sometimes the exact location of the problem is difficult to determine since the steps are sequential. In other words, if you have a problem with storing, the error will be reflected in retrieving and using. Even worse, if the error occurs early in the sequence, everything that follows will be flawed, just as it was with the Leaning Tower of Pisa. Shortly after its completion in the 1170s, the tower began to tilt because the engineer who designed it misjudged the soil's density.[3] No matter what he did to correct the mistake, the lean increased. The same thing happens with information processing. If we can identify the step where the error occurred, we not only better understand the senior moment but also gain insight into its prevention.

Impaired Attention

The brain is wired to make sense of the information presented to it.[4] One technique it uses to accomplish this is "grouping" or classifying what it encounters. For example, a box of round objects that vary in size, color, and texture is placed in front of you. Instead of just viewing everything inside as separate objects, the brain identifies them as similar enough to be in a group labeled "balls." Some neuroscientists consider the brain's ability to categorize similar to what a computer does when categorizing objects, events, and even emotions.[5] But comparison can take us just so far. The world's fastest supercomputer requires twenty-four million watts of power to operate, but our brain only requires twenty and is a hundred thousand times faster than a computer.[6]

Another significant difference between our brain and a computer is "fact-checking." The brain never quite "fact-checks" the way a computer does. If it did, many senior moments would not be created. For example, you write an email with a specific address, and your Internet server "decides," whether to accept or reject it based on criteria such as:

1. Does this email address have all the necessary components?

2. Is this address on a sender's "do not accept" list?

3. Is this address on a blacklist?

When it finishes the analysis, you then receive a message such as "email sent," "no such address," or "forbidden address."

Nothing is this straightforward when the brain processes information. For example, someone you love says, "You aren't sensitive to my needs. You never listen." The brain compares the incoming data with its memory of experiences and beliefs and responds by thinking *Okay, I know what the words mean, but is that true? Is that what I remember doing? Am I capable of being insensitive?* If this is new information, the brain stores it with minimal distortion for future use or adds a filter, such as "emotions," that colors it. But, if the information is not new or is a modification of what has already been stored, the brain sees it through additional filters that include experiences, beliefs, and needs.[7]

Here is an example that many of you have experienced. Imagine entering a noisy restaurant where you must scream to be heard by the person sitting next to you. The waiter comes to your table and explains the special of the day in a soft voice. What you hear is just a jumble of sounds, with a barely audible "mesquite grilled." *Wonderful,* you think, *it's my favorite—rack of lamb.* "I'll have the special," you say, recalling the taste and smell of your best meal. Twenty minutes later, the waiter delivers a plate of liver—a food you despise. To avoid embarrassment, you eat the entree, gagging on each bite. Your dinner companions often retell this story as an example of a humorous senior moment when, in fact, it was a problem of impaired attention caused by noise.[8]

Misunderstanding

Misunderstanding can occur because of content or the form in which the information appears. For content, think about a time when you had difficulties using a new software program. You read the manual at your desk in a quiet room with no distractions and thought you understood how to install the software. You began the installation by recalling the instructions, following each step exactly, and praying the program would work. If it did not, you would have to contact a customer service representative with a difficult to understand accent or ask your granddaughter for help. Neither choice was appealing.

When the program refused to run, you reluctantly chose your granddaughter's condescension as the lesser of two evils. She came to your aid, and, in a few minutes, the program was running, and she had another "Grandma story" to tell friends. Unbeknownst to you the instructions were an inadequate translation from Japanese to English, which did not affect your granddaughter's understanding since she was "computer savvy." The family chuckled that "Grandma is stuck in the stone age." However, the source of your embarrassment was a misunderstanding error, having nothing to do with your cognitive ability or reluctance to enter the twenty-first century. The fault was the software company's reliance on someone with a limited understanding of English to translate a technical document from Japanese.

Misunderstandings can also occur because of the form in which the information appears. I chose to learn Spanish when I was in my sixties. I sat attentively on the first day of class and waited for the teaching to begin. Señorita Marten entered the room and stared at twenty other senior citizens who were enthusiastic about learning a new language. After a few minutes of excruciating silence, she slowly said in heavily accented English, "Some people think Spanish should be learned by teaching it in English. I am not one of those foolish people. Today is the only day you will hear me speak English. For the remainder of the semester, only español!" My attention was fine; I listened and watched what she wrote on the blackboard, but I still could not understand Spanish because of the form Señorita Marten insisted on using.

Incomplete or Inaccurate Storage

Researchers believe the placement of memories is complicated, with bits stored in various parts of the brain waiting for reassembly into a unified picture.[9] We do not know how the brain stores memories, but we think it is in the form of chemicals that reside in various places.[10] When called upon, these data nuggets reassemble and form a montage of experiences and emotions. For example, a few people are talking about their favorite fishing spots, and someone mentions Henry's Fork, a legendary river in Idaho. My brain goes into a high-speed search for anything connected with the phrase "Henry's Fork." It finds pieces of information spread throughout billions of neurons, such as its location, the fish I caught, the smell of blossoming thistle, the sound of gentle ripples, and the sight of thousands of insects emerging from crystal clear water and making my body their new home. My brain assembles everything into a unified picture, and I re-live a day in one of the most peaceful places I ever fished. My recollection would be very different if I could not remember its location, forgot the feel of the insects, the fish I caught, etc.

Inaccurate Retrieval

Inaccurate retrieval is expected as we age.[11] We are told we should accept a faulty memory as an inevitable part of aging. And when we have difficulty retrieving significant events, a well-meaning person might say, "Of course, you remember," assuming retrieval is no more complicated than turning on a light switch. But it is far more complex. Let us assume that your memory of an event five years ago was accurately stored. At a party, someone asks you to recall the heated discussion you observed at that event. Your description of the encounter dismays your partner, who also was present at the event. She thinks, *that's not what happened. How can he get it so wrong?* There was no intention on your part to exaggerate or misinform, rather, the fault lies with your brain's physiology; it rarely retrieves a memory as it was originally stored.[12] In the 1960s TV series *Dragnet*, Sergeant Joe Friday implores witnesses to stick to the facts when telling him what they saw. "Just the facts, Ma'am," is a line in almost all 276 episodes. The characters' inability each week to exactly retrieve what they stored kept the show's audience entertained for eight years.

Inaccurate retrievals can also be understood by looking at how children learn a language. A young child's brain is like a sponge, ready to absorb every drop of water it contacts. However, what it stores can never be more than the model presented. I often worked with parents who did not understand why their child's speech contained so many articulation errors. When I did a language sample, I found that the model these parents used was full of "baby talk," which they felt was endearing but presented a less than accurate model of speech for the child's brain to absorb.[13] If their child primarily heard an imperfect model of English, that would be the best they could retrieve when speaking. So it is with memory. If something distorts an experience, the brain records the distortion rather than an accurate rendition.

Inaccurate retrievals also result from a person's history. Investigators used magnetic resonance imaging (MRI) to compare what goes on in the brains of several people as they listened to the same story.[14] The MRI findings showed differences across subjects in terms of which parts of the brain become active. The results might explain why I cried watching the final battle scene in *Les Misérables* and the person sitting in front of me fell asleep.

Similarly, it may explain why you have a senior moment, and your friend does not.

Recent findings suggest that every time an event is recalled, it changes. Not a lot, but just enough to slightly deviate from what really occurred.[15] The process is similar to the children's "telephone game," where a child whispers a statement to the next child in line. By the fifteenth retelling of the story, the original innocuous message about the weather has been transformed into something scandalous that happened in the teachers' bathroom. Your brain will go through a similar process each time you recall an event or tell the same story.[16] It is a physiological response ripe for creating a senior moment.

Other nefarious things can throw a roadblock in front of retrieval, like a lack of sleep, multitasking, and noise, among others.[17] When I was counseling, I knew a miserable night's sleep would interfere with my ability to recall, late in the fifty-minute session, what my client shared with me at the beginning of it. If I were thinking about a personal problem while conducting a counseling session, the thoughts would interfere with remembering the concerns my client expressed in the beginning of the session. It was just as problematic as the construction noise coming from the street.

Inappropriate Usage

Many of our "inappropriate usage" senior moments involve behaviors that are accurately retrieved but not appropriate for the context in which they are used. For example, I play a Peruvian wooden flute called a *quena* and hoped to jam with indigenous musicians on a trip to Peru. Before leaving, I practiced several short musical phrases called "licks." They are a series of notes that sound good when played together. Licks are inserted throughout songs and provide embellishments to basic melodies. While accomplished musicians know hundreds of licks, my repertoire consists of less than twenty.

After my wife and I planned our trip, I spent months memorizing the licks and practiced retrieving each perfectly. When we arrived at the train station for Machu Picchu, I saw a few musicians playing for tourists and asked if I could join them; they graciously agreed. Although I retrieved each lick perfectly, I did not use any of them appropriately. The crowd still heard the melody but knew something was wrong. I'm sure they figured that whatever it was, it was coming from the old guy with Harpo Marx hair. On the upside, my wife had another embarrassing story to share with our friends.

BAD ACTORS

Let us say your brain is accurately attending to incoming information, understanding its meaning, storing everything accurately, and using it ideally. Are you out of the woods for having a senior moment? Not quite. The information processing system can function just as it should, but still be susceptible to bad actors: your psychology, physiology, and data overloads.

Psychological

Everybody sees the world through an amalgam of "stuff." For example, my favorite movie is *Field of Dreams*, a film I still cry through every time I watch it. It is also the film my wife slept through, my daughter tolerated watching, and my son, after listening to my reverence for it, thought I was hopelessly nostalgic. How could such different reactions come from watching the same movie? It concerns how our needs, values, and experiences massage information.

I never objectively watch *Field of Dreams*. I see it through the strained relationship between myself and my father, my unfulfilled childhood aspiration of playing first base for the Yankees, and my college social activism. I am not just watching a critically acclaimed movie, but rather the story of my life. My wife and adult children are mystified by my sobbing at the end of the film.

They view my inexplicable emotional behavior as—you guessed it—a senior moment rather than the confluence of my experiences, needs, etc.

Physiological

The brain's cognitive ability is sensitive to physiological changes.[18] Those changes are influenced by illness, disease, drugs, hydration, nutrition, and sleep. For example, a family was to gather for a special dinner. The daughter-in-law worried about meeting her father-in-law's culinary expectations. To make a good impression, she made a complicated Moroccan dish called chicken bastille. The night before the dinner, she slept for only four hours. Her insomnia could have been related to a new medication or dehydration following a ten-mile run. Her dream of impressing her father-in-law ended when he gagged on the first bite. Instead of a half cup of sugar, she had used a half cup of salt. Her father-in-law gloated that although he was twenty-five years older than his daughter-in-law, she was the one having a senior moment when, in fact, changes in her brain's physiology were what caused the error.

Data Overload

There is a wonderful scene in the movie *Amadeus* where the composer, Mozart, finishes playing a new piece for Emperor Franz Joseph. The young composer, ready to gloat over another successful musical accomplishment, asks the emperor how he liked it. The emperor mulls over the question and responds that it was fine, except it had too many notes for him to attend to. Just like the emperor's, your brain may often face situations that produce a data overload. What happens when the brain is overloaded? It will either ignore new data, dump old data, or slow down, much like your computer does when your RAM reaches a critical point.

Regardless of the pathway the brain takes to relieve the pressure, the overload will cause information processing problems and create conditions for a senior moment.

CHAPTER 3

A Very Short Primer on Memory

*The human brain has one hundred billion neurons, each neu-
ron connected to ten thousand other neurons. Sitting on your
shoulders is the most complicated object in the known universe.*
—MICHIO KAKU[1]

THE THEORETICAL PHYSICIST MICHIO KAKU'S PRICELESS GEM
about the power of the brain is exemplified every time you go into
a restaurant. You read the menu, decide what you want to order,
return the menu to the waiter, and go back to an animated discussion with friends. Ten minutes later, the waiter returns and asks
for your order. Without any hesitation, you say, "spicy noodles."
How did you remember your selection? You did not write it down,
nobody coaxed you, yet there it was, "spicy noodles."

Memory is a phenomenon as mysterious as the universe.
Some, like Michio Kaku, believe even more so. Everything we
do, every thought we ever had, is produced by the human brain,
but exactly how it operates is an unknown. What is exciting for
researchers is that the more they probe its secrets, the more sur-
prises they find.[2]

Although nobody knows precisely how we retain information,
speculation is rampant.[3] An explanation for why you remembered

your dish is that your brain understood what the written words on the menu meant, you selected an item, and your brain placed the information in an area where it could be quickly accessed (short-term memory) if needed. Sometimes this ability is flawless. For example, the waiter forgot your order and returns to the table, and you repeat it. At other times, it can lead to a senior moment; the waiter returns, and you cannot remember what you chose. This is a memory lapse your friends find amusing, since only ten minutes elapsed.

Think of memories as three-dimensional pictures with sounds, tactile sensations, and odors. While some are fleeting, such as the name of someone you just met, others seem to be epoxied into your brain. Here is a short experiment demonstrating the brain's mysteries. Turn on a favorite news show without looking at the screen and listen to a newscaster's voice, one you have often heard. Now with your eyes closed, imagine the shape of the person's face, the color of their hair, and even the expression you imagine they have. Your accuracy of the familiar newscaster's image in your brain will probably be high. You may not recall all of their features, but enough that the match is undeniable. But how did you do it?

WHAT WE KNOW AND DO NOT KNOW ABOUT MEMORY

You probably have seen television gurus and authors suggesting you buy a $39 memory kit, or a memory pill based on a proprietary formula. The items, they claim, will restore your brain to the power it had twenty years ago and add ten points to your I.Q. However, at the bottom of the screen, in an unreadable font, are the qualifiers. How many of their promises come from what they *know* and how many from what they *believe*? How much of their pronouncements are based on solid research? There are many things we inherently know about memory, things you do not need scientists or authors to confirm. But many others remain a mystery, such as why repeating a simple direction increases the probability you will remember it ten minutes later. What we assert about memory can be based on **(1) direct evidence, (2) observation-based guesses, (3) injury-based guesses, or (4) intervention-based guesses**.

Direct Evidence

While direct evidence is a hallmark of research, when it comes to memory it has the fewest findings and constantly changes as technology improves. For example, in the past, scientists thought that once brain cells were damaged or died, new cells could not be generated. Recent research shows that new neural cells can be created, even in Alzheimer's patients.[4] We also know through dissections that the brain's wiring is present at birth, and the connections between the billions of neurons are chemical and electrical.[5] Especially pertinent for senior moments, we know that the brain breaks up experiences into sensory units (touch, vision, hearing, and smell) and stores them in various areas, with much redundancy (e.g., duplicate information may be stored in more than one area.) [6]

Observation-Based Guesses

Most of our knowledge about memory comes from observations.[7] B. F. Skinner in the 1960s championed observation as a scientific method. He viewed the brain as a black box.[8] He and other behavioral psychologists maintained that although we see what goes into the brain and what comes out, what happens inside is a mystery—the infamous black box of psychology. Many of our inferences about memory are based on observable behaviors, not knowledge of the brain's physiology. There is nothing wrong with making inferences as long as they are not assumed to be direct evidence.

Injury-Based Guesses

Researchers often infer conclusions about memory from behaviors following an injury.[9] They compare the workings of a healthy brain with one that has been damaged, hoping the differences *may* provide indirect evidence of the damaged area's responsibilities. For example, a stroke victim is given a hammer and asked what it does. Despite knowing its name, because of their injury they cannot explain its purpose. From this, researchers will extrapolate that the damaged area of that patient's brain is responsible for attaching a function to objects. Many scientists object to using a damaged brain to infer how an undamaged one works.[10] They rightly argue that the range of damage can be so variable that it is possible to get contradictory results even though the site of lesion in two brains can be identical.

Intervention-Based Guesses

Another source of memory speculation is based on the positive effects of a memory improvement strategy, such as those found in this book. For example, a client randomly placed their car keys in different coat pockets, resulting in their searching for the keys every time they needed them. I developed an intervention strategy that required my client to place their keys in the same pocket for one hundred days. At the end of the experimental trial, without thinking, they consistently dropped them in the same pocket. Based on the strategy's outcome, I concluded that with consistent practice, the brain can learn to perform some behaviors automatically.

TYPES OF MEMORY

To add to the mystery and confusion about memory, terms such as "short-term" and "long-term" are tossed about as if everybody agrees on their meaning. Nothing can be farther from the truth. Unfortunately, these inconsistencies appear in literature and advertisements for supplements and "brain-training" programs. Whenever possible, I will refer to behaviors rather than types of memory. When that is impossible, below are my definitions for sensory memory (iconic memory), short-term memory, long-term memory, sequential memory, and working memory (executive function).

Sensory (Iconic) Memory

Your brain, like a camera, captures everything to which it attends, similar to a video camera that records everything within the lens' focus. This endless recording process is called sensory or iconic memory. It occurs whenever we see, smell, hear, and touch.[11] The image or sensation we experience in each of these senses momentarily stays in place before it moves to an area in the brain thought responsible for creating short-term memories.[12] For example, you smell barbecued ribs and hot dogs as you walk by a local park with a friend. Although you move past the grills surrounded by large groups of laughing people, the image remains as you and your friend discuss what both of you just saw; a remembrance of your happy childhood days spent in the park near your home.

Short-Term Memory

The image from the park is vivid for a short time until the brain sends it for later use to an area responsible for short-term memory. But what is short-term memory? You would hope that since we are dealing with neurology, there would be a universal definition everyone could use to avoid confusion. Unfortunately, there is not.[13] Some researchers define short-term memory as impressions that last between twenty and thirty seconds.[14] Others are more generous, asserting that short-term memory is everything you experience until you fall asleep, which is when the brain consolidates them into long-term memories.[15] Researchers frustrated with the slice and dice approach, discard time as a method for classifying memories and instead focus on where memories live.[16] To add to the confusion, some neuroscientists insist that the amount of information the brain stores differentiates short- from long-term memory—a little for short-term, a lot for long-term.[17] When the term "short-term memory" appears in this book, it refers to information stored until sleep when the brain consolidates memories—such as the barbecue in the park—into retrievable vignettes (long-term memory) following sleep.

Long-Term Memory

Defining "long-term memory" is fraught with the same type of problems as describing "short-term memory.[18] Some researchers maintain that long-term memory is anything that occurred moments, hours, or decades ago.[19] With no sharp time demarcations, if you accepted this definition, you would constantly struggle with deciding if a memory is short- or long-term. In this book, short-term memories are consolidated by the brain into long-term memories following sleep.

Sequential Memory

Sequential memory comes into play with behaviors that require multiple steps, with each new step dependent upon finishing the prior one.[20] It is the type of memory necessary to complete a multi-step project, like putting together your grandson's bicycle or remembering why you went to the kitchen. Senior moments involving sequential memory occur when you either cannot remember a previous step, such as the third step in a six-part assembly of a cabinet, or why you decided to stop working in your home office to walk to the kitchen.

Working (Executive Function) Memory

"Working memory" or "executive function" refers to the brain's ability to process, hold, and manipulate information that resides in sensory, short, sequential, and long-term memory.[21] Working memory (or executive function) is illustrated by what a cook must do to make an omelet (Some neuroscientists make a distinction between "working memory" and "executive function." For our purposes in this book, we will ignore the subtle differences.) To accomplish the task the brain searches for information in its long-term memory, such as the importance of cracking eggs without getting pieces of the shell in the mixture, the need to butter the pan, etc. Other bits of information will come from short-term memory, such as where you put the eggs after today's shopping, and others involving the sequential steps necessary to go from cracking eggs to eating the omelet. Problems in working memory are often the first sign of dementia.[22]

Part II

Strategies

In reality, strategy is actually very straightforward. You pick a general direction and implement it like hell.
—Jack Welch[1]

We look for quick fixes for problems—plastic surgery for wrinkles, affairs to rekindle feelings of youth, or a new Maserati to create an image of wealth. But neither a $100,000 car nor a facelift will help you remember where you left your keys. However, strategies will. The term "strategy" describes an approach that can solve more than one problem and, as the late Jack Welch, former chair and chief executive of General Electric, wrote, points you in a direction. For example, instead of treating specific behaviors (e.g., how to stop losing keys, how to stop forgetting your cell phone, etc.) I taught a client a strategy—structuring the environment to minimize misplacing anything important.

Strategies tell you *what* to do. However, knowing what to do does not automatically translate into applying that strategy to the prevention of a specific senior moment. For that, we use "methods." For example, slowing down is a strategy for most types of senior moments, but you will need to drill down for ways to apply it. The ways or methods in this next section will always be in italics and bolded. At the end of each method section is an "action summary." Sometimes a method will be found under only one strategy, such as **prioritizing** for combating inertia. But other methods, such as **meditation** are important for two different strategies—focus and sleep. And still others, like **visualization**, will help with many strategies. You might also find that even though a method is only found under one strategy, for your circumstances, it may be helpful in implementing numerous strategies. You might wonder if each method is rigidly tied to a strategy. No. For example, although **mindfulness** can help increase focus, it also may be important for attitude adjustment.

CHAPTER 4

Slow Down

Be slow in choosing a friend, slower in changing.
—BENJAMIN FRANKLIN[1]

BENJAMIN FRANKLIN PACKED MUCH WISDOM INTO FEW WORDS. In the above quote, he encapsulated one of the most basic principles of change: Do it slowly if you want to be successful. Few people want to hear that to change anything significant in their lives, they should do it slowly. We want financial security in a year, enlightenment in one week, and perfect health yesterday.

Unfortunately, as we age, "quickness" is not our friend, since the time required to accurately process information increases.[2] Neurology is not as accommodating as imagination. For those of us approaching our twilight years, the slower the speed, the less likely we will have a senior moment—regardless of what we are doing. Numerous studies have found that the quicker we do something as we age, the greater the possibility of errors.[3]

Doing something quickly often results in taking in more data than we are neurologically ready to assimilate. That condition was graphically displayed in one of Monty Python's most infamous skits. Mr. Creosote, a gluttonous diner, stuffs himself with multiple orders from the menu. With each serving, he grows larger, his body engulfing his chair. The waiter comes to his side and offers him a mint. Mr. Creosote moans, "Not one more thing," but the waiter insists. "Oh Sir, it's only a tiny little thin one." The man replies, "I can't eat another thing. I'm absolutely stuffed." The waiter insists until the man recants, eats a small mint, and, literary explodes. Just as with Mr. Creosote, with data overload, your brain arrives at a point where it can no longer function well. It will not explode but relieves pressure the way a boiler's relief valve does. As the pressure in the boiler rises to a dangerous point, the valve opens, and steam escapes. With your brain, data escapes, is ignored, or becomes distorted. There are methods to prevent these problems while **(1) listening, (2) reading, and (3) doing**.

LISTENING

You are driving to an unfamiliar area, your GPS is not working, and you ask a stranger for directions. You have difficulty understanding what they are saying because of their accent—one that is new to you. You ask them to repeat the directions and they do at the same speed they said them the first time. You smile, thank them, and wonder when you will be able to find someone whose speech is easier to understand. Instead of driving five minutes to your destination, you circle, as I did, in an unfamiliar area for an hour, unable to find the street with the name you thought the stranger said. A frustrating moment like this and similar events are often labeled as senior moments, but they result from a speech perception error.

What is a speech perception error? The best way of understanding it is by examining what happens when you are trying to get help from a customer service representative. We begin with the representative's greeting: "Hello, my name is Shaun. I hope you're having a great day. How can I help you today?" The auditory signal is first detected in your ears as mechanical energy—sound waves, which are converted to electrical impulses in the cochlea (inner ear), sent to the brain via your nerves, then converted into meaningful words.

But let's say there is a problem with the transmission. Shaun, the customer service rep, reads from his script, but some words are unintelligible to you. You hope if he speaks louder, the problem will be corrected. You make the request, and after apologizing, he compiles. But you are astounded when you still cannot understand some words. No matter how loud he speaks, the words are still distorted. Sometimes a specific reason for the hearing problem can be found, but usually, it is idiopathic—a $20 word meaning we do not know why.

Most likely, the problem has to do with age-related difficulties in recognizing one or more parts of a spoken message, such as articulation (how a word is said) or features of a word's sounds (phonemes).[4] The problem becomes most evident when trying to understand accented speech.[5] Possibly the aging brain becomes more restrictive in matching what it hears to what it stores.[6] The ability to accurately perceive spoken words is a problem that affects most people as they age, some more than others.[7] These problems do not happen all at once, nor with all words. It develops slowly and is often detectable only years after it began.

Currently, we cannot reliably determine if listening senior moments are caused by information coming in at a speed the brain can no longer handle or if they are due to a signal distortion problem. Fortunately, we do not need to make a differential diagnosis to prevent senior moments caused by either. You can use the following methods for both: **(1) ask the speaker to slow down, (2) introduce a speed bump, (3) prepare, (4) create a written framework, and (5) simulate the interaction.**

Ask the Speaker to Slow Down

How often have you misunderstood the words someone is saying in your native language? You may have experienced this problem watching British movies even though your first language is English. When I was younger, I could watch English movies for hours and never miss a word. However, as I aged, I found I had to be more attentive to understand what was being said, and sometimes, even if I focused, I could not understand who did what to whom. And even if I did understand everything, I was so exhausted at the end of the movie I vowed never to watch a British film again without English subtitles.

People sometimes mistakenly label senior moments caused by speech perception problems as xenophobia, which is "extreme, intense fear and dislike of customs, cultures, and people considered strange, unusual, or unknown." I had a client who complained to friends about customer service representatives with foreign accents. Many believed racism was the basis of his complaints. "You know, Jim's got prejudices," they would say, mistaking a speech perception problem for a racially motivated comment.

Asking the speaker to speak slowly is a good method, but what is a good target rate for the speaker to use to prevent your senior listening moments? When I was doing therapy, I strove to keep my speech under one hundred words per minute, a rate that facilitates understanding for clients even if they didn't have a speech perception problem.[8] However, this skill, which took years to develop, left me exhausted after each session, since I was asking my brain to do something unnatural. Getting someone to speak slowly so you can understand them can be difficult because their brain wants to return to its normal speech rate. Strangely, your request that people speak slower will often result in them speaking louder. Not a helpful response since loudness only minimally increases accuracy.[9]

Why is slowing down an effective method regardless of whether the problem is caused by a hearing loss, a speech perception problem, or something related to cognition?[10] Think of two gears whose teeth must mesh perfectly for a device to work. The interface will be clunky if they are out of sync—even by a millisecond. Metaphorically, that happens when information is coming in at a speed your brain cannot handle. If you give the brain an additional few milliseconds to digest the incoming data, it will be better prepared for the information flow.

Despite your pleas to the customer service representative from India to slow their speech rate, and their honest efforts to do so, their rate will often ultimately drift back to its neurologically determined speed within five minutes.[11] In fairness to out-of-country customer service employees, their companies are clueless that fast rates frustrate customers with listening problems.[12] Some representatives are actually encouraged to speak faster so more clients can be served.

While it is difficult for speakers to keep their speech pace at a desired slow rate, it is always worth asking them to try.

Introduce a Speed Bump

Speed bumps effectively force speakers to slow their rate by restricting the flow of information. It is similar to the reduction in water pressure that occurs when a hose goes from the faucet to the tiny drip opening in the feed line. Speed bumps will give your overworked brain a chance to rest. Start with less intrusive ones, like asking for a restatement of what the speaker just said. For example, a client complained to me about a supervisor's marathon lectures criticizing the unit's poor performance. They said listening to the supervisor was like reading a three-page paragraph without punctuation. The comments came at such a rapid rate the supervisor was in the middle of the fourth topic before my client digested the first. By the end of the forty-five-minute conference, my client said their brain felt like a freeway entrance at rush hour.

The next time they had a meeting with their supervisor, they used a gentle speed bump, asking for a restatement. "Let me see if I have this straight. You believe the people I am supervising are not meeting your goals, right?" Instead of a delay long enough for my client's brain to catch up, the supervisor said, "Right," and quickly moved on to other topics. My client decided to use a more disruptive method, this time saying, "Excuse me, but I need to use the bathroom." While this was not as polite, it was definitely more effective.

> *When speakers cannot or will not reduce the rate at which they are speaking, introducing a speed bump that forces them to slow down can give your brain a momentary respite.*

Create a Written Framework

Advanced preparation is a simple but effective method for increasing comprehension and preventing senior listening moments.[13] Creating a written framework to map incoming information allows you to pigeon-hole what you hear during a presentation.[14] For example, imagine you will be attending a meeting where management will explain a new project. You know the presentation will involve:

1. The project's name

2. Who will be in charge

3. When it will begin

4. How much it will cost

5. Your role in the project

You can enhance your understanding and memory of the presentation by writing the five topics on a sheet of paper with space to jot the information down as the presentation progresses.

Creating a framework into which you can drop information during a speaker's presentation will enhance your ability to understand and remember what was said.

Simulate the Interaction

Simulations are methods in which one uses structured practice to prepare for an event.[15] Examples are political candidates' practice sessions for debates, surgeons learning procedures by operating on corpses, and sculptors who work with a clay model before striking their first blow on a fragile block of marble.

Simulations train the brain to become more attentive.[16] We think simulation works because it develops a structure in our memory that mirrors the target activity.[17] If the key elements of the simulated activity are comparable to the target activity (i.e., topics, length of time, speech, etc.), your understanding and recall accuracy will improve, eliminating a major cause of listening senior moments.[18]

Create scenarios similar to what you will hear at a presentation, such as a rapid speech rate, long utterances, no breaks between sentences, etc. The more similar the simulation is to the real activity, the less likely a senior moment will occur. If you can find a willing partner, enact the presentation. During simulations the brain goes through a learning process that is similar to what happens in artificial intelligence experiments, where the software's knowledge base increases with each successive action.[19]

If you cannot find someone to simulate the speaker, listen to speakers on TV or on the Internet and take notes as you would during a work presentation. Start by watching a presentation of a person speaking at a rate of speech you find comfortable. If you are successful in understanding their presentation, move on to someone speaking slightly faster. With each success, find a slightly faster speaker, ending with someone who speaks faster than the person for whom you are preparing.

Simulations also work by enabling you to better understand accented speech. You can also focus on the type of speech the speaker will be using, not just the rate. If you are moving or traveling, say, from New York to London or San Francisco to New Orleans, you can prepare by watching films or videotapes where speakers use the target dialect. Since your brain is continually processing information, you can train it to expand acceptable parameters of words by repeatedly listening to a speaker with an unfamiliar accent. Each time you listen, the brain gathers new information or learns to make more accurate distinctions between different pronunciations of the same word.[20]

With repeated listening, the brain's evaluation becomes more accurate, and less effort is necessary to focus on pronunciation during a live presentation. This frees more cognitive energy to assess content rather than dwelling on whether you heard "Sarah" or "Sahara."

Why use films or videotapes for training rather than audio recordings? Audio signals with visuals are easier to understand than examples without visual contexts.[21] So, unless you plan on keeping your eyes closed during a presentation or circumstances prevent you from using visual stimuli (e.g., phone conversations), always train with a video component. If your target speaker is someone you will interact with regularly, record their speech, then listen to it multiple times.

Simulations that are able to include most or all of the important elements of a target activity prepare you better for what might be a stressful presentation. The more familiar you are with a speaker's speech pattern, the more likely you will avoid comprehension errors that could lead to a senior moment.

Reading

A person told friends that life was discovered on the moon. When they asked where he learned that, his response was, "I read it in the *New York Times,* of course!" Yes, the *New York Times did* have a story about the moon, and life, but it was just a speculation on whether life could have existed a billion years ago on the moon. His friends used the misinterpretation as an example of "Charlie losing his mind." From that point on, whenever a group member's voracity was questioned, the person's response was "the *New York Times,* of course!" a comment everyone thought humorous except for Charlie.

Yes, his "facts" appeared in a newspaper known for scrupulous vetting, but Charlie had skimmed the article while sitting in a noisy bus on the way to work. All that distraction made comprehending and retaining details difficult, resulting in Charlie's senior moment. Such reading senior moments can be prevented by using any of the following methods that directly or indirectly slow the speed of incoming information: **(1) reduce the reading rate, (2) eliminate scanning, (3) subdivide the contents, (4) pay attention to the beginning and end of units, (5) keep it quiet, and (6) change the format.**

Reduce the Reading Rate

A computer-savvy client tried to learn a new software program in a short amount of time. In the past, he had been able to breeze through more complicated software programs in minutes. After failing to understand the program, he assumed the problem was in its instructions. It was not. The errors resulted because his reading speed exceeded the rate at which his brain could accurately comprehend. My client's frustration and failure stopped when instead of trying to learn the whole program in fifteen minutes, he slowly read the instructions over one hour. The simplest way of reducing the possibility of having a senior reading moment is to slow down.[22] If you have problems intuitively slowing your reading—many people do—read aloud. The process of audibly reading reduces your rate automatically, thereby giving the brain additional time to process visual information.[23]

The faster you read the more likely you will misunderstand. The more you misunderstand, the greater the possibility of having a senior moment. Slow your reading speed by at least 25 percent.

Eliminate Scanning

Scanning places pressure on the brain by asking it to simultaneously comprehend current and forthcoming words.[24] The more you can focus on the words you are reading, the greater the probability that your reading will be error-free, and therefore senior-moment-free. While scanning is a skill essential for musicians reading sheet music as they play, it can be disastrous for readers who lack violinist Isaac Stern's genius.[25]

A technique to eliminate scanning and stay in the present is to place your finger under the word you are reading and move it along at a pace slower than the one you use while reading silently. Another technique to limit scanning is to use an index card placed underneath the sentence. The card puts a visual bracket beneath the material and improves reading comprehension. I taught this technique to stroke clients who have reading problems and clients whose deficits stem from normal aging.

If you are focusing on what you are reading and what comes next, you are dividing attention between the present and the future. Splitting attention increases the possibility of misunderstanding. Focus just on the word you are reading.

Subdivide the Contents

A senior trying to learn all the features of his new car became frustrated when he tried to quickly link his phone to the car's hands-free program in fifteen minutes. He began to experience success when he stopped reading at the end of each individual section, summarized in his mind what he had just read, then continued on to the next section. This strategy allows your brain to catch up with the barrage of data a book or article forces it to analyze. You can also slow the overall pace of your reading by taking short breaks between sections, to rest your brain or write a few summary sentences.

Natural breaks already exist in good writing: a sentence, a paragraph, a section, a chapter. If authors are savvy on how people comprehend, they will insert strategic breaks throughout the material, giving readers time to "catch up." Unfortunately, some writers ignore punctuation, and others believe punctuation does little other than slow down texting. It does slow down inputting but compensates by helping comprehension, especially in seniors.[26] Punctuation omissions become fertile ground for confusion in seniors. Here's another quick experiment you can try. Read the following memo that a supervisor sent to her employees:

> We will be going over material today gathered by our sales unit. The number of suggestions will be based on Jeff and George's research over the past three months. Tomorrow we will implement the first three suggestions, then next week, the remaining ideas will be implemented unless the sales figures don't warrant it. I will be making those decisions the following week after Jess analyzes the data using our new computer software. If you can't implement the ideas, then you will need to make an appointment to discuss your problem.

Now contrast his list of ideas in the original memo with the same one that is segmented.

We will be going over material today gathered by our sales unit.

The number of suggestions will be based on the research that Jeff and George did over the past three months.

Tomorrow we will implement the first three suggestions.

Then next week the remaining ideas will be implemented unless the sales figures don't warrant it.

I will be making those decisions the following week after Jess analyzes the data using our new computer software.

If you can't implement the ideas, then you will need to make an appointment to discuss your problem.

Which version is easier to comprehend? Which version do you think would be easier to remember?

For printed material, insert your own breaks using a red marker to subdivide. If what you are trying to read is on the Internet, insert breaks before you print the document. I use this strategy with clients who have comprehension difficulties. You may think this needlessly adds time to your reading, and it does add some, but only minimally. On the upside, you will immediately notice that your comprehension improves, and you will need fewer passes to understand the document.

Use the natural breaks (or insert your own) within reading passages as an opportunity for your brain to catch up with what you are asking it to do.

Pay Attention to the Beginning and End of Units

The beginnings and ends of well-written material (sections, chapters, paragraphs, etc.) contain the most important ideas. By highlighting them, you decrease the likelihood of misinterpreting the main idea. Excellent writers will labor over the beginning and end of what they are writing[27] because they understand openings will often set the reader's mind for the entire section, and endings serve as a bridge to the next unit.[28] Spend more time on lead-ins and endings than the middle.

Here is an excerpt from my book, *Loving, Supporting, and Caring for the Cancer Patient*.[29] Only the beginning and ending sentences of a paragraph appear in this excerpt.

Beginning Sentence

Our minds often do a balancing act with the truth on one side and necessity on the other.

Ending Sentence

The butcher didn't think adding a few cents to the bill was dishonest but rather a necessity for keeping the doors of a marginal business open.

If you just read these two sentences, you probably would conclude that the missing content contains ideas related to how we do things we are not proud of out of necessity. Now read the entire paragraph below.

Our minds often do a balancing act with the truth on one side and necessity on the other. An example is the "butcher's thumb," a common practice before prepacked meats became available in the 1960s. The butcher would place his thumb on the edge of the scale while weighing a piece of meat, adding a few ounces to the total. He knew what he did was wrong but justified the dishonesty with an economic pressure argument: "A few pennies won't make a difference to my customers. At the end of the month, it can mean the difference between keeping my shop open or closing it." A personal need to believe in something—just as the necessity of a butcher's thumb—changes what's real. The butcher didn't think adding a few cents to the bill was dishonest but rather a necessity for keeping the doors of a marginal business open.

Although the other 105 words provide more information, just the first and last sentences are sufficient to know what I tried to convey. Is highlighting a substitute for a complete read? No, but the technique focuses on the "meat" of an article or book and provides transitions to other ideas. I taught this method to a client who had difficulty participating in her book club's discussion. Although she always read the book, her comprehension errors often resulted in comments other members thought were "off-the-wall." By using the highlighting method, her comments became spot-on.

Yes, you say this could work with well-written documents, but what about the others where structure does not appear to be a part of the writer's arsenal? You may have to keep that yellow highlighter in hand as you go through the entire piece.

You can streamline the information in a document by focusing on those elements that contain the most important information.

Keep It Quiet

How often while you read do you listen to the TV or try to compensate for the material's boredom by listening to music? You believe your reading material's complexity is so minimal that you can listen and read at the same time. I hate to be the one who dispels this notion, but you cannot—at least not accurately. Although noise affects comprehension in children the most, seniors' comprehension is not immune.[30] So, if your senior moment involves reading, turn off the music or TV and find a quiet place to read with minimal noise.

Accurate reading comprehension can be affected by any form of noise. Keep your reading environment as quiet as possible.

Change the Format

Although not strictly a speed issue, changes in the font size and spacing may influence the flow of information. How often have you squinted when reading an article, even when using reading glasses, eventually skipping over portions of it or putting it down? The effects of font size and spacing on comprehension are inconclusive.[31] However, you do not need a research study to guide you, just change the font size or spacing to see the effects. Find a short article on the Internet and experiment with changing the font size to between eight and sixteen. Also change the spacing and the bold feature. You might find there is little difference, but do not be surprised if a slight change in the size of the font, a greater separation in the lines of print, or shading an important sentence dramatically affects your comprehension.

Experiment with changes in an article's or book's font. When you find what's most comfortable, use it as the standard for modifying reading material on your computer or tablet.

DOING

A friend insisted his reaction time was just as good at age seventy-six as it was at forty. His wife was less delusional. She complained that her husband had been ignoring the decline in his information processing abilities since it began in his forties. As he whizzed through lanes on the highway, narrowly missing cars, his passengers, including me, prepared for the afterlife. My friend's neurological changes could not be reversed by wishes. He was not forty any longer, would never be forty again, and, if he did not change his attitude and driving, he never would see seventy-seven. While you cannot go back in time, you can use methods to compensate for slower reaction times.[32] To reduce senior moments related to doing, you can **(1) reduce the speed of what you are doing or (2) add time to complete the activity**.

Reduce the Speed

I learned to type in high school. Speed minimally affected my accuracy when I was young. I was as accurate at forty words per minute as I was when approaching eighty words per minute. Now, when I am in a rush and try to type fast, my computer screen becomes populated with strange errors that make me rhetorically ask, "Where did that come from?" When I start seeing many of these gremlins, I know I am trying to make my fingers work faster than my brain can match. The simple solution? Slow down my typing speed. You can use this speed-reduction method on all senior moments that arise from physical behaviors. Continue whatever you are doing, just do it slower.

You do not have to be exact in how much you slow down. I worked with a client who loved woodworking but did everything, including using power tools, at a dangerous speed. While he still had all of his fingers, his wife feared the eventual loss of digits. She insisted he sell his power tools and take up a less dangerous hobby, like gardening. He adamantly refused. I suggested a compromise: Stretch out the amount of time he allotted for each step in a project. For example, measure twice instead of once before cutting. Instead of the quick moves of a saw blade, something he was proud of, I suggested he carefully and slowly move the blade over the board. Instead of completing a project in one day, take three days. Did the methods work? My client still has ten fingers, and his wife no longer prepares to call 911 whenever he goes to his workshop.

By slowing down the speed of what you are doing, you enable your thoughts and behaviors to sync.

Add Time to Complete the Activity

Have you noticed that it takes you longer to get ready for an outing today than it did last year? To prepare dinner? To make decisions? There is nothing unusual about this as we age. If we accept these inevitable changes, life becomes more relaxed in the second half of our lives than if we rushed through it. However, our high-tech, youth-centric world is not very accommodating to slowness. The result? We rush and create the perfect storm for a senior moment.

Several years ago, a friend invited my wife and I to a formal event where well-known dignitaries would be present, some of whom would be introduced to us. While I was always early for appointments, my wife was notorious for being late—for everything. It became so predicable that our friends would always adjust our meeting time by fifteen minutes. As the time approached when we needed to leave our house for this formal event, my wife still was not dressed. My attempt to rush her by hovering and constantly ticking off the time did little other than annoy her and increase the time necessary to get ready. As a result of my impatience, I created her senior moment. When we arrived at the event, my wife realized that although both of her shoes were black, they were different.

Assume it will take you longer to complete something than you anticipate and add time to every activity.

CHAPTER 5

Combating Inertia

There is only one way to eat an elephant—a bite at a time.
—BISHOP DESMOND TUTU[1]

ALTHOUGH THE IMAGE OF SOMEONE EATING AN ELEPHANT WILL be humorous to some and offensive to others, it does highlight what can be accomplished by not "biting off more than you can chew." Think about something you have done for many years that you have never challenged. You may not like what you are doing. Still, it has been in your behavioral or idea inventory for so long it is as comfortable as an old slipper. That is what Newton would call "inertia," his first law of motion states *a body at rest will remain at rest unless a force acts on it*. Although his observations and laws were for physics, Newton could have been a change expert if the discipline existed in the 1700s!

As important as Newton's First Law is to understanding physics, it is equally important in understanding why you may avoid changing personal and social behaviors that lead to senior moments. Take, for example, a common type of senior moment: forgetting names, numbers, and events. In the past, your memory allowed you to hold ideas and appointments in your head without writing them down. Now, as your short-term memory develops problems, you stubbornly believe your recall ability today is as great as it was twenty years ago—even when you repeatedly forget to attend meetings, pick up dinner, or buy a present for your grandchild's birthday.

Behaviors such as these will not magically vanish through wishful thinking. Behaviors and ideas, just like physical objects, need a nudge to move. You may recognize that something has to change if you want your embarrassing senior moments to cease. Still, you have no idea what could serve as a nudge. Two methods can help move you from reoccurring senior moments to a life without them: **(1) making change easy, and (2) making change rewarding**.

MAKING CHANGE EASY

When I was thirteen years old, my parents forced me to practice the accordion in my room above their grocery store. "An hour a day," my teacher instructed. "Don't you want to be the next Dick Contino on the *Lawrence Welk Show*?" he added as an extra incentive. My mother did, so she diligently monitored my practicing as she cut lunch meats for customers while they swayed to my rendition of "The Beer Barrel Polka." My teacher expected me to go from zero practice time to one hour daily in one gigantic step. It was so punishing; I still cringe every time I hear an accordion.

Unfortunately, I forgot the importance of making change easy with each new instrument I attempted to learn. Instead of applying the lesson from my accordion days, I allowed my ego to run rampant and adapted the philosophy that if I just practiced enough, I could become the next great soloist in the San Francisco Symphony. As failures accumulated with the violin, dulcimer, banjo, piano, and resonator guitar, I thought the instruments were the source of the problem, not how I attempted to learn them. My efforts with these instruments were viewed by my friends as examples of musical senior moments. The joke was, "Stan doesn't play musical instruments—he collects them."

When I began playing wooden flutes in my sixties, I finally realized that my style of practice had caused past failures, rather than anything inherently tricky about the instruments. Instead of adhering to the "practice till you drop" maxim, which left me wondering why I continued, I started with twenty minutes, three times a week. At the end of each session, I was hungry for more practice time. Instead of giving in to that feeling and extending my practice, I let it carry over until the next scheduled session, which I began as if I was reuniting with a friend rather than being forced to spend time with my third-grade teacher. I added five minutes to each session every week, eventually reaching one hour. It was a lesson in making change easy, not only for learning an instrument, but for any behavior I wanted to change.

The struggle to leave a life plagued by senior moments to one devoid of them should require almost as little effort as not changing.[2] We often think of change as involving monumental moves, applied with gruesome determination necessary to achieve big goals—precisely the wrong thing to do unless you are a masochist. Your attempts to change will be more successful if you relax, sit back, and make the change as easy as possible. You can move from having senior moments to a life without them by implementing three methods: **(1) select small goals, (2) arrive at your destination in tiny steps, and (3) experience many tiny successes.**

Select Small Goals

When we select goals, our natural tendency is to choose ones that are life-changing or mind-boggling. While laudable, this tendency almost guarantees needless failures. A kinder method is to divide that memorable goal into ones that are easier to achieve. Behavioral psychologists call these "successive approximations."[3] Put more colloquially, the *select small goals approach* is equivalent to Bishop Tutu's eating the elephant one bite at a time. The lesson was lost on a client who wanted to stop repeating stories in all situations, all the time. A laudable goal, but so comprehensive it was doomed to failure before he even began. So, instead of starting with this global quest, I suggested he focus on specific situations. His first goal was not to repeat stories at home with his partner. The second was to not repeat stories with friends when playing tennis, and the third to not repeat stories at parties.

Although it is wonderful to have big goals, the path toward achieving them will be so littered with failures you may give up on achieving the goal.

Arrive At Your Destination in Tiny Steps

I remember watching a cognitively disabled adult learning how to wash dishes in a restaurant. His trainer would meticulously break down each of the activities into small sequential steps. For the first he prepared the plates for washing. The second involved racking the plates according to size and on and on. The trainer explained each step, and then the dishwasher practiced one step until it was mastered, then moved on to the next.

Watching the laborious learning process was excruciating for the chef. This was something she felt should require no thought at all. "After all," she said, "you don't hire a skilled craftsman to wash dishes." As she continued her preparation for the next meal service, her annoyance slowly transformed into admiration for her new dishwasher and the trainer. After one hour, the dishwasher had learned the same tasks it would have taken two minutes for someone without a cognitive disability to learn, but with a major difference. Not only had he learned his assignment flawlessly, but he performed each aspect of the task perfectly.

While chopping lettuce, the chef had a revelation. If dish-washing could involve as many steps as she witnessed, what about her own cooking activities? She began looking at various tasks, such as salad preparation, sauce making, plate presentation, and grilling. She was amazed that each of these activities she had been performing for fifteen years was really a series of activities, some of which she performed flawlessly, while others were less than adequate. For the next month, the chef diligently worked on each skill with which she was dissatisfied, eventually developing food presentations that resulted in her and her restaurant receiving rave reviews.

I used the same approach with a client who had difficulty understanding books discussed at her book club. After reading ten pages she would forget what she read on the first few. Instead of participating in the group's discussion, she remained silent for fear that her comments would be interpreted as foolish. However, she felt my proposed method was too laborious to analyze the book. She suggested an alternative approach of simply dividing the book into its logical divisions: paragraph, page, and section, and summarizing each unit in writing.

It is not as elegant as the one I proposed, but it was more acceptable to her. And that is the approach you should use with all of the methods in this book. If it is not acceptable to you, disregard it no matter how much I say you should not.

Learning a new behavior that will replace a senior moment should be easy. The probability of success is increased by dividing a behavior into small units.

Experience Many Tiny Successes

How often have you assumed the British "stiff upper lip," where you decided to struggle to accomplish a goal? Maybe that involved painting your entire house over the weekend or installing a software program you are sure was designed to frustrate you. Your painting project was a disaster since you did not allow enough time for the paint to dry before putting on a second coat. And although you were able to install the sophisticated software program, without understanding some advanced programing it remained unused in your computer along with seven other pristine programs.

Researchers have found that people are more successful when they divide their larger goals into smaller, more attainable ones rather than squaring off with undivided ones.[4] For example, I have always wanted to play the Irish tune "The Mason's Apron," a complex piece for flute with notes that seem to fly out of the instrument. If I tried playing the piece at its intended speed in one gulp, I would be lost and wonder if I should have continued with the accordion. But could I learn it by playing each bar slowly until I mastered it, before going on to the next one and repeating the process? Although I am only up to the sixth bar after months of daily practice, I have continual successes rather than failures.

We are so accustomed to lauding big successes that we diminish the importance of smaller ones. Yet, it is the series of many minor successes with few failures that are better for our progress and our souls than multiple failures on the way to achieving "the big one." A big success following multiple failures does not outweigh the positive psychological effects of a series of small wins with few or no losses.[5]

If you routinely forget names, instead of having "do not forget any names, ever," as your goal, try to choose the name of just one person to remember. Your first step might be to use that name three times every day for a week. You might wonder how something that easy can result in not forgetting a name. Think about the importance of "foundations," whether that involves golf, cooking, knitting, or playing a musical instrument, to mention just a few. Proficiency in each of these activities rests on mastering foundation skills, as does the ability to remember names. Although you believe saying someone's name three times a day in context is meaningless, your brain disagrees. The simple exercise of using one name three times a day for a week lays the foundation for remembering other names in various situations.

As a speech-language pathologist, I have witnessed the reluctance to "think small" with clients who wished to change something fundamental about themselves or their children. Stutterers wanted to be completely fluent immediately. Parents of disabled children wanted non-disabled kids to accept their child on the first playdate. People who suffered strokes wanted to have comfortable conversations days after their neural insult. These clients wanted to achieve their goal in one step and immediately, which is understandable but counter to what research tells us about how change is achieved and sustained.[6]

How often have you been asked to summarize something? It could be a movie you watched, a book you read, or an event in which you participated. The request to "tell me about the movie," is so broad that you become confused, and your answer becomes less than cogent, leaving your questioner wondering if you really saw the movie or read the book at all. Succinctly summarizing a book was a problem a writer faced when the editor of an online journal asked her to write a 1,200-word review. She had completed assignments like this in the past in just an afternoon. But now, she felt her analytic skills had slipped—not much, but enough that she was producing articles whose quality was being questioned by her editors.

I taught her a more systematic approach involving divisions. There are various ways of dividing a "whole." One that we used was to first divide the book into characters, themes, plot, conflict, and resolution. Then, each category was further divided until no more divisions made sense. For example, characters were identified as antagonists, protagonists, or neutral. Themes were labeled as either "primary" or "secondary."

The smaller the sequential units, the easier it will be to achieve a goal. The easier a goal is reached, the quicker a senior moment is prevented.

Making Change Rewarding

Human beings are rational—at least most I know are. We yearn to do activities and have experiences that make us feel good. Psychologists refer to this phenomenon as "reinforcement." We also try to avoid those activities that are punishing. Given a choice, I doubt if anyone would choose to put their hand on a hot stove rather than eat a delicious piece of chocolate.

However, the powerful role reinforcement can serve in preventing senior moments is often overlooked. An example of the effects of reinforcement was a man who perpetually lost objects in his house. He would lay them down when he no longer needed them and not remember their location. He did not consider it a major problem since they would eventually be found. However, keys and wallets were special. He was reinforced to remember where his keys were by being on time for appointments when he didn't have to search for them. Having a wallet when he left the house meant being able to purchase his morning latte.

As children, most of us experienced two forms of behavior control. Punishment for doing something inappropriate, and reward for doing something that pleased our parents.[7] Unfortunately, punishment is often the "go-to" strategy to change behaviors. As a child, your parents probably required you to do things you did not want to do, such as cleaning your room. When you asked why, the response may have been "because I said so." Adults, as well as children, need a positive reason for doing something, whether that's clearing dishes from the dinner table or retrieving past events more accurately.

If the motivation is to avoid punishment—whether you are a child or a senior—the new behavior will be fragile, a lesson I learned when I enrolled in a karate class to gain flexibility. The instructor came into the dojo and faced twenty adults who, like me, were excited about learning karate. As we began our first stretching exercise, he yelled, "No pain! No gain!" and proceeded to tell us that this exercise would be painful—just like the other ten he would be asking us to do. For the next three weeks, I forced my legs to move in ways God never intended. By the fourth week, only three people remained in the class—and I was not one of them.

Changing from a life filled with senior moments to one devoid of them should not be punishing. If it is, the probability of you doing the necessary actions will be as remote as me remaining in the karate class. So forget about using punishment to eliminate your senior moments. You should not be doing the activities because "I said so." They should be enjoyable and rewarding. Design your activities to include at least one of three types of reinforcement: **(1) intrinsic, (2) extrinsic, or (3) extraneous**.

Intrinsic Reinforcement

Intrinsic reinforcement occurs when the act of doing something is enjoyable. One example is a man whose cooking was the source of senior moments. For dinner parties he always insisted on preparing four or five courses. By the time he was finished preparing the third, guests were arriving. The joke was if you were going to Gene's for dinner, be prepared to have your salad at midnight. What had been a joy for him became drudgery. By simply reducing the number of courses to two, Gene made preparing food once again intrinsically reinforcing to himself and his guests who were now able to finish dessert by 8:00 p.m.

Intrinsic reinforcement is a potent tool for change since it taps into the enjoyment you experience from doing an activity. If you cannot find anything intrinsically reinforcing to prevent your senior moment, look for something extrinsically reinforcing.

Extrinsic Reinforcement

Extrinsic reinforcement occurs from the completion of an act. A client did not find any exercises I designed for remembering names intrinsically reinforcing. If I insisted he do them, I knew his efforts to eliminate these senior moments would stop. However, he took pleasure in retrieving and using the names of relatives. He was willing to do uninteresting activities to experience the joy of successfully retrieving his nephew's name during a short telephone conversation.

> *When there is nothing intrinsically or extrinsically reinforcing about a task, look for extraneously reinforcing elements.*

Extraneous Reinforcement

Extraneous reinforcement is reinforcement that is neither inherently a part of the act nor its completion. Some people consider it a last-ditch effort to prevent senior moments when no other form of reinforcement is possible. Money is the best example of an extraneous reinforcer—it works to keep someone at a tedious job and learn an unenjoyable behavior.

For example, I designed a strategy for a client who lost objects in his house. The first step was to locate specific places where those objects would "live," this required him to clear some areas and create new "homes" for them. There is nothing enjoyable (intrinsic reinforcement) about the activity. He was required in the second part of the strategy to consistently place the items in their assigned spots. Again, nothing enjoyable (extrinsically reinforcing) here. So why continue? He gave himself a point every day if he put the objects in their designated places. After a certain number of points, he treated himself to a decadent plate of ice cream (extraneous reinforcement).

Sometimes to prevent a senior moment, you might have to do activities that give you no enjoyment in their doing or completion. By rewarding yourself for successfully completing them, you will move forward in your elimination of the senior moment.

CHAPTER 6

Patterns

To understand is to perceive patterns.

—ISAIAH BERLIN[1]

ISAIAH BERLIN'S ASTUTE OBSERVATION BECAME THE THEME OF the 1993 movie *Groundhog Day,* in which Bill Murray's character wakes every morning in Punxsutawney, Pennsylvania, and repeats what he did the previous day. What follows are identical responses from the town's citizens and its most famous resident, "Phil," the groundhog, who can predict spring. Eventually, Murray's character begins to understand that events will not change if he does not alter his behaviors. While he was right that something had to change, it was not a behavior—but a pattern.

A pattern is a set of linked behaviors that usually results in a predictable outcome. They are everywhere, found in the movements of the smallest insect to the rotation of planets; from chord changes in Bruce Springsteen's "We Are Alive" to Mozart's transition of movements in "Requiem." You can see them in how termites construct their dwellings in California, New Jersey, and Texas despite never exchanging blueprints, and how identical air currents form in Oklahoma, Germany, and Asia before becoming tornados. Patterns also can explain why a factory worker in

Savanah, an executive in Detroit, and a baker in San Francisco repeatedly forget their wallets when they leave for work in the morning.

Because patterns group behaviors into chains, they allow your brain to do many things that help its functioning. One is to "coast," which is to engage in repetitive activities such as making your daily cup of coffee without focusing on each step. When your brain coasts during a routine activity, it can direct more attention on what may be new or important. Coasting allows the brain to take a break from being attentive. Take my daily pattern, which has changed little in forty years.

1. wake up at 4:00 a.m.

2. have coffee

3. visit the bathroom

4. check my emails

5. feed the dogs

6. write

It is as if every morning I press a button at 4:00 a.m. and the sequence begins as it did for Murray's character. The pattern is so strong that if I do not do one of the behaviors, my brain screams, "Hey, this is not what I am used to. Get back on track!" You've probably had a similar feeling when you left your house, knew you forgot something, but had no idea what it was. Think of a pattern as a set of dominos lined up, waiting to begin an inevitable march when the first one is tipped over. To understand the strength of a sequential pattern, you do not have to look any further than a troubled relationship. You can almost always predict when it is about to go off the rails. Rarely is it just because of a single behavior. For example:

Domino 1. You forget an appointment with a friend.

Domino 2. She tries to make you feel guilty.

Domino 3. You defend yourself aggressively.

Domino 4. She stops taking your phone calls.

Domino 5. You reunite and wait for the pattern to resume next month.

To change a pattern such as this or any other ones that negatively affects your life, you can: **(1) disrupt old patterns or (2) create new patterns**.

DISRUPTING OLD PATTERNS

A man joined a group of people at a party in the middle of a conversation where he heard sympathy being expressed for a drug user not at the party. He chimed in without knowing what the full conversation was about.

"Drug users are such losers," he said. "I don't understand why we don't just jail them."

Before he finished saying his last words, a woman in the group burst into tears and left the room. The remaining people explained to the man that the woman's daughter recently committed suicide after multiple rehab failures. Although truly sorry for what he had said, he attributed it to coming into the conversation after it started—something he thought was forgivable, something that could be corrected by a simple apology. His friends, however, saw it differently. In the past, he often expressed controversial ideas without understanding the issues. His ingrained pattern was to:

1. Listen to a discussion.

2. Make an unequivocal judgment.

3. State his position forcefully.

4. Respond aggressively to every questioning comment.

This pattern occurred with grocery store clerks, customer service representatives, and even with people he was meeting for the first time.

Sometimes patterns are so entwined that they remain as hidden as the contents of Skinner's black box. Unfortunately, we search for a behavior that causes a senior moment rather than looking for a reoccurring pattern. If you lose your glasses, you probably also lose your keys, cell phone, etc. Should each of these senior moments be considered a stand-alone event caused by different things, or is there a pattern of behaviors that ties them together? In most cases, you will find a unifying pattern created by an information processing error.

Patterns establish themselves in your brain so firmly they become automatic. For example, I have been driving for more than sixty years. Although I think I am observant when driving, I know most of my reactions are automatic and contained within patterns. For example, when I see a yellow light, I start to slow down, judge the distance between my front bumper and the rear bumper of the car ahead of me, and finally, I constantly adjust the pressure on the brake until I come to a stop. My first domino is the yellow light. That is the beginning of a pattern I do not want to disrupt. But there are others I *do* want to change or eliminate, such as not listening as well as I should at parties, on the phone with friends, or when asking for directions from a stranger. This can be done by **(1) eliminating triggers, (2) lessening emotions, or (3) erecting a wall to stop the progression**.

Eliminating Triggers

Our brain is loaded with patterns that have been imprinted on it. Some neuroscientists cite the ability to create and recognize patterns as one of the most essential characteristics of the human brain.[2] Every pattern has a trigger. For example, you decide to do something to stop the daily loss of your glasses. You want to determine if there is a sequence of events that leads to it. It does not take you long to discover the culprit. You sleep through your clock's alarm every day for at least fifteen minutes. What follows is rushing through your morning ritual of selecting clothes, making coffee, gathering materials for the day, and finally putting your reading glasses into your pocket. You realize that the triggering event is sleeping past your 6:00 a.m. alarm. By eliminating that trigger, you should be able to avoid losing your glasses. You decide to move your alarm clock to the far side of the room, so you will need to get out of bed to turn it off.

> *Since your senior moment is caused by a trigger acting as the first domino in a chain, the senior moment can be eliminated or disrupted by removing the trigger.*

Lessening Emotions

A pattern's strength may be related to the emotions experienced when a behavior begins. For example, a new approach to the Golden Gate Bridge contained a dangerous curve. Although a sign warned to slow down to thirty-five miles per hour, the first time I drove there, I was too distracted to see it. When I realized the danger, I was traveling at sixty-five miles per hour and had to brake as hard as I could to avoid careening off a concrete buttress. Seven years later, although I approach the curve at twenty-five miles per hour, I still have those feelings of panic.

There are various ways of lessening the effects of an emotion, and most involve some form of psychotherapy. One that you can do on your own is called systematic desensitization.[3] Systematic desensitization diminishes an emotional response by repeatedly confronting or experiencing it. I reduced my anxiety when approaching the curve by going over the Golden Gate Bridge every day for weeks. The gut feeling I had the first time I almost had a tragic accident has not gone away, but my anxiety when approaching the bridge has reduced.

Eliminating an emotional trigger is more difficult than a physical one. Systematic desensitization is effective but may still leave traces of the pattern.

Erecting a Wall to Stop the Progression

It may not be possible to eliminate a pattern just by purging a trigger, especially when the trigger has friends. When trying to stop smoking in college, I eliminated what I thought was the trigger—a cup of coffee—yet I was still unsuccessful at stopping smoking. I realized my nicotine addiction was so strong that just eliminating coffee was not sufficient to stop the pattern, which began by holding a cup and ended with smoke streaming into my lungs. I needed to give my desire to stop smoking an advantage over my nicotine addiction's entrenched pattern. It was like trying to shift the balance on a seesaw from an overweight bully on one end and a skinny kid on the other.

The solution was to add weight to the weaker side. So, whenever I went for a cup of coffee, I would look at a picture of someone dying of throat cancer, examine the ugly gray sputum I saved when I coughed upon waking, and look at the long flight of stairs I needed to climb after leaving my house. The pattern was not immediately disrupted, but I have not smoked cigarettes in more than fifty years.

The first step in changing a behavior is stopping the progression of the pattern that is creating it.

CREATING NEW PATTERNS

Sometimes a senior moment can be prevented by just disrupting an old pattern, especially one whose grip on your brain may not be that strong; a pattern that has minimal emotional overlays; few associations; or, because of limited repetition; is still fragile. But usually, it needs to be replaced by a pattern that reinforces the new substitution. This can happen by **(1) creating triggers, (2) repetition, or (3) memorization.**

Creating Triggers

Just as triggers are crucial for starting a senior moment pattern, they are effective in creating its replacement. A man wrote the wrong amount on his checks so often his adult children insisted they review them before he mailed them. He hoped to stop his embarrassment and the family's stories by carefully writing each number, believing that attention to writing the numbers alone would correct the problem. Unfortunately, incorrect dollar amounts continued to appear. The electric utility company could not care less since his checks were always significantly more than the amount owed. The IRS, however, was not amused when they received a check for $208.00 instead of one for $20,800.

Check-writing errors in the past tended to occur when the man wrote them in the evening after an exhausting day, following a glass of wine. After receiving a threatening letter from the IRS and admonishment from his adult children, he realized he needed to change the pattern that led to his mistakes rather than just giving more attention to the actual writing of the dollar amounts. Feeling refreshed, whether in the morning when he woke or anytime in the day, signaled to him that it was a good time to write checks.

Every pattern begins with a trigger. Create and strengthen a trigger that can initiate the pattern.

Repetition

Watch Stef Curry when he sets up for a midcourt shot during a game. His movements are identical to what they are in practice before the game, during training sessions, and probably during the off-season. The time that elapses between him getting into position and shooting averages an amazing 0.4 seconds—hardly enough time to think about what his body needs to do to score.[4] Yet Curry is the all-time three-point leader in the history of basketball.[5] Why? My guess is that it's because of repetition and, yes, a whole lot of talent. On average, Curry shoots at least five hundred shots from various positions on the court before every game.[6] There are no reported figures on non-game practice days, but you can assume it is at least five hundred.

With repetition, a behavior becomes more automatic, requiring less time to think.[7] Although you may not want to become a basketball star known for shooting three-point shots, you may want to have a flowing conversation without having to constantly think about remembering names. That will happen if you can make the behavior automatic. Think about a skill you learned. Most likely, the more you did the behavior, the more "glue" was applied to it, firmly affixing it in your memory. For example, when I am making bread, there is a pattern suggested for how to knead the dough so that more gluten develops. I have made so many loaves of bread that the four-part kneading behavior is now automatic. Neuroscientists speculate that repeatedly doing a behavior creates automaticity, which is a ten-dollar word meaning that the brain does not have to "think" once a pattern is initiated, it just kicks the first domino.[8]

But repetition alone is not sufficient to make a behavior automatic. Intention must also be involved. Intention is simply being highly aware of what you are doing as you do it. Without intention, the behavior may still eventually become automatic, but with it, the process becomes more efficient and more quickly developed.[9] For example, a golf instructor showed me where I should bend my wrists in the swing. He told me to practice for fifteen minutes, and that he would return to assess my progress. I did exactly as he instructed, but I was distracted by a scandalous conversation taking place next to me.

Sometimes I hit the ball perfectly, but other times when my neighbor's description of his sexual conquests became lurid, I was a danger to everyone on the driving range. When the instructor came back, he saw that my swing was inconsistent. He told me to continue the exercise, but this time, he would yell, "now!" when I approached the release point. This simple cue enabled me to intentionally bend my wrists, embedding the pattern in my memory with a better outcome than practicing the swing while listening to the sexual exploits of the person next to me.

> *The more you repeat a desired behavior with intention, the more likely it will form into a pattern that is retained and easily retrieved in a sequence.*

Memorization

Memorization is a strange phenomenon whose value is often underestimated. We scoff at its rote nature rather than seeing its importance in creating new behaviors to replace undesirable ones.[10] I asked a chorus member of the San Francisco Opera how he could sing the lyrics of more than forty operas without knowing the languages in which they were written, other than English. He explained that a common practice for singers is to memorize one bar at a time regardless of the language in which the opera was written. He would repeatedly sing a single measure until he could recall it easily and perfectly. When that goal was met, he worked on the second measure with the same goal of perfection. Then the two measures were strung together and practiced. He repeated this sequence until his lines were committed to memory.

When he retrieved his part during a performance, he did not feel he had to concentrate on recalling the words but could focus on how to sing each note. Memorization is a valuable method for preventing many types of senior moments.[11] For example, memorizing the names of people you will meet at a dinner party can be very successful.

Memorization can create ideal conditions for instituting a pattern that will replace a senior moment, and it is the mental equivalent of practicing a behavior.

CHAPTER 7

Challenge Your Brain

A scientist is just a kid who never grew up.
—Neil DeGrasse Tyson

Do you remember when you were the child Tyson describes above? The kid who found everything intriguing, from how ants built a colony to why fire burns fingers? Like most young children, you probably tortured your parents with an endless series of "why" questions they could not answer. And if they could answer one question, you pummeled them with a follow-up "why," never stopping until they walked out of the room or told you to go out and play. With age you became an adult who questioned less and accepted more. This is not necessarily bad for social cohesion, but it is antithetical to what may be required for preventing senior moments.

The adage, "use it or lose it," applies to buttressing your brain's ability to prevent senior moments. Think of your brain's activity as falling on a continuum. On the lowest end is the passivity present when watching reruns of your favorite television show. At the upper end of the continuum is trying to allocate your paycheck for bills in a way that avoids creditors sending you to collection. There probably is no sharp boundary between beneficial activities and those that have no impact on preventing senior moments other than giving your brain a respite.

Even though there are no scientific studies comparing the cognitive benefits of watching reruns to listening to a lecture on derivatives, it should be obvious which activity would be more beneficial for intellectual growth and the development of new neurons. I am not saying there is no place for passive entertainment. It is essential to give the brain breaks to prevent it from crossing a threshold and experiencing exhaustion.[1] So do not feel guilty about watching one rerun as a break from preparing a tax return. However, binging on *Judge Judy* will not be helpful when you are trying to retrieve a memory.

As we grow older, we lose neurons and synaptic connections because of illness, disease, or just age-related conditions.[2] In the past, most neurologists thought that once a cell died, a new one could not replace it, nor could new connections be generated between cells. But research has shown that not to be the case. Finding that new neurons (neurogenesis) and new synaptic connections (synaptogenesis) can be developed even in the brains of people having dementia transformed what we thought we knew about the brain.[3]

These results are mind-boggling! It is like looking at a washed-out road and realizing there are alternative ways of arriving at your destination. And how does one do that, you might ask? By challenging the brain with activities that are **(1) creative or (2) cognitive**.

CREATIVITY

Creativity should not be considered the province of luminaries. It is a process accessible to everyone from gifted artisans to your boring uncle Ralph who watches TV for twelve hours a day. Creativity is universal. It requires the same skills, whether you are the famous Michelin three-star chef Alain Ducasse creating new dishes for the Dorchester Restaurant or a recent Haitian immigrant in a Brooklyn take-out joint trying to replicate their mother's recipe for baked pork shoulder. And what are these skills? Bryan Goodwin and Kirsten Miller suggested the answer in a 2013 article. They hypothesized that creativity required six skills.[4]

1. Providing multiple answers based on the available information

2. Constant analysis of what is being created

3. Willingness to redraft and start over again

4. Ability to engage in complex and creative problem-solving activities

5. Ability to combine convergent and divergent thinking

6. Willingness to ask "what if?" questions

As you may notice, end products are not mentioned in any of the skills—they are irrelevant. My sculptures are laughable compared to ones done by professional sculptors, my musical compositions are only slightly better than the tunes hummed by my seven-year-old granddaughter, and my modifications of tried-and-true recipes often result in inedible dinners. Although it would be nice if people praised my creative efforts, that is not why I do them. These activities have the potential for creating new neural connections that can preserve my cognitive ability or at least slow down its deterioration.

Since the value of creativity has nothing to do with an end product, you can be creative even if you believe what you produce is terrible. For example, I enjoy tying artificial flies for fishing. I can follow the directions precisely for making a "woolly bugger" or modify parts of the instructions to create a unique pattern. Granted, I'll probably catch more fish with the established pattern, but by making modifications to the pattern, I am exercising my brain. Even for the "Goldberg Woolly Bugger," each of Goodwin and Miller's skills are required:

1. Providing multiple answers based on the available information:
   Should the body color be black or brown to match the lake?

2. Constant analysis of what is being created:
   If the body gets too fuzzy, I will need to clip the legs shorter.

3. Willingness to redraft and start over again:
   The chenille is encroaching on the hook eye. Time to start over.

4. Ability to engage in complex and creative problem-solving activities:
   If the wind comes up, I'll have to fish the pattern differently.

5. Combining convergent and divergent thinking:
   I know how the pattern should move, but will the fish see it the same?

6. Willing to ask "what if?" questions:
   If I bounce the fly off the bottom, how will it move?

COGNITION

As I mulled over Goodwin and Miller's six skills, determining if they appeared in each of my creative activities—they did—I realized that they also were present in any activity I identified as cognitive. I use the same skills when I write, work on finances, try to learn how to build a deck, and a multitude of other cognitive activities.

The similarities that exist for cognitive and creative activities were explored on a PBS series called *A Craftsman's Legacy* hosted by Eric Gorges who travels across the United States to gain insight into craftsmanship in the twenty-first century.[5] The one question he asked each legendary craftsperson was, "Is what you do a craft or art?" which to me translates into a cognitive or creative activity. Although some felt forced to choose, most settled on "both," lending credence to the notion that the skills necessary to be creative are similar to those essential for cognitive tasks.

Why are these skills important? By developing and using them, one can structurally and functionally change their brain, resulting in increased cognitive performance and well-being.[6] Your brain benefits when you spend thirty minutes deciding where to plant the zinnias instead of watching the news, thinking about how to lay out a stone walkway instead of being lulled to sleep by the *Wheel of Fortune*, or planning a dinner party rather than watching a cat video on YouTube.

COGNITIVE CREATIVE ACTIVITIES

"Creative" and "cognitive" were once thought to be two distinct types of activities generated from different parts of the brain: cognitive activities from the left hemisphere, and creativity from the right. However, recent studies on brain plasticity indicate that cognition and creativity are found on both sides.[7] Additionally, if an activity is creative or cognitive, the brain uses up to 50 percent more oxygen than needed when engaging in a more "couch potato" activity such as watching reruns of sitcoms.[8] It is oxygen, according to some research articles, that improves cognition in the elderly.[9]

Instead of labeling your activities as either "cognitive" or "creative," ask yourself if they require Goodwin and Miller's six skills. My suggested activities involve cognitive reasoning and creative deliberation, and they all require the six skills listed by Goodwin and Miller. Don't expect results tomorrow. Just as muscle strength takes time to develop after years of idleness, so does improved memory and reasoning abilities. But you will immediately experience a delightful side benefit: Engaging in creative activities allows you to stay in the moment, temporarily blocking out the daily grind of life. Not bad for something so easy to do and beneficial for your brain and soul.

Below I have listed twelve types of cognitive/creative activities that research says will aid in generating new neurons and synaptic connections. There is no rank order of their potential benefits nor recommendations for how long to do them. However, you can use the maxim:

1. Spend more time on these than on passive activities.

2. Do at least one every day.

3. The more time spent doing these activities, the greater the results.

And even if you do not see any benefits immediately, think how much better you will feel looking at a fired clay pot with your design instead of ticking off the number of *National Geographic* episodes you watched that day.

Modify Existing Activities

Every morning, I drive the same way to the park where I walk my dog. There is nothing creative about the routine. But what if I made a game of how I would get there? For example, I could roll dice each day, and the number that came up would determine how many blocks I drove in the opposite direction before heading to the park. Although it may appear silly, changing how I get to my arrival point is creative, requires cognitive effort, and if I wish to make it there before my dog pees in my car, I will need to use Goodwin and Miller's six skills.

> *Even slight modifications of set routines require the brain to shift from what was old and comfortable to something creative and analytical.*

Add Something New to a Routine

Instead of changing a routine, it might be easier to add a new element. For example, when watching your favorite TV drama, pause it every ten or so minutes, and predict what will happen when you resume watching. Who will Olivia on *Law and Order* accuse of the murder? Will Rachel uncover another shocking fact about politics? It makes little difference how correct your predictions are. What is essential is that you are activating the six skills.

> *Adding one or more new elements to a pattern disrupts a "knowledge set" the brain thought it knew. It will require the brain to compare and contrast the old with the new pattern.*

Engage in an Activity that Constantly Changes

Every day I spend between two and three hours sculpting wood or stone. With each chipping away of material, I need to decide where I will make the next cut, how much to take off, and how the amount will affect my overall design. Most art activities involve the same type of constant changes.

> *Constant change, while disruptive, requires the brain to stay alert, preparing it for changes that may occur in various activities.*

Begin New Activities Regularly

The best example is learning a new language. Everything is fresh: the meaning of words, syntax, and pronunciation. You are constantly matching words in the new language with their English equivalents and then coordinating them with the muscles required to speak them. A similar cognitive/creative process occurs when you improvise a melody on an instrument or compose a poem.

The beginning of new activities has a similar effect on the brain as activities that constantly change.

Listen to Music Differently

When we listen to music, it is rare that we focus on its structure. We listen to be entertained, to relax, or rejoice. I am no different most of the time when I listen to Billy Strayhorn's "Take the A Train." With the first notes I am bobbing on a crowded subway car going from Kennedy Airport to Brooklyn. A lovely break from writing an essay on compassion. But sometimes, I will listen to the chord changes and see if I can guess where the chord sequence will go and how the melody will move through the piece.

You can do the same by choosing a song or a movement from a symphony or sonata that is not too complicated. Try to isolate the repetitive rhythm of a bass, the sequence of notes played by the lead guitar, the violinist's integration of her solo into the orchestra's arrangement, etc. As you listen, you will notice you are using Goodwin and Miller's skills.

Listening to music analytically is an experience very different from listening for pleasure. It can be done while working around the house, riding in a car, running, etc. Regardless of the setting, it can be a stimulating activity for the brain.

Exercise Your Brain with Puzzles

Who would ever think a simple jigsaw puzzle could be a mental callisthenic for preventing senior moments? Jigsaw puzzles require the brain to engage in visual perception, construction, orientation, visual scanning, flexibility, perceptual reasoning, and episodic memory.[10] When using puzzles, start with the one that can easily and quickly be completed. You may believe it would be embarrassing if your six-year-old grandson saw you playing with a puzzle more appropriate for him than an adult. And it might be if the goal was to complete the puzzle—but it is not.

To complete even a young child's puzzle, you will need to *visually perceive* what is being depicted. Flex your *construction skills* by connecting each piece. Develop the ability to *orientate* each piece into a position to accept another one. Your eyes will constantly be *visually scanning* all pieces to find ones that can be connected. You will learn to be *flexible* when pieces you thought would fit do not. Your *perceptual reasoning* will be strengthened when you look for pieces that fit, and lastly, as you scan the pieces on the board, your *episodic memory* will have to move your impressions to short-term memory.

Wow! An unbelievable number of benefits from just putting together a simple puzzle depicting Old McDonald's Farm. Once you feel comfortable with a simple puzzle, move on to one slightly more complicated. Finally, when you have established your puzzle "chops," take on the challenge of a one-thousand-piece puzzle.

The value of puzzles is underappreciated. To complete even the simplest one requires all of Goodwin and Miller's skills and others.

Work on Creative Writing

Teachers in grade school sometimes ask children to create a story. As a fourth grader, I loved that type of assignment. It allowed me to envision distant places, loving and despicable characters, and the outcomes I wanted for an ideal life. Other than recess, it was my favorite school activity. What I did not realize was that besides being enjoyable, it contributed to my cognitive development since it required me to make decisions, organize, create goals, plan, translate, and review.[11] Precisely the type of activities that keeps the brain engaged, alert, and prepared to avoid senior moments.

Who would ever think something so enjoyable that we do as children could be so beneficial for us as seniors?

> *Creative writing taps into most of the cognitive benefits of puzzles and adds to the element of fantasy. Start with a story that has specific characters, location, a beginning and ending, and a limit of five hundred words. As you feel more comfortable, become adventurous in your writing, reduce the number of set items, and strive to be the next Toni Morrison or Ernest Hemingway.*

Challenge Yourself with Video Games

It is Christmas morning, and you cannot wait for your four-year-old granddaughter to open your present to her. You struggled to find just the right game; something that held your attention for hours when you were a child. In the remotest corner of a shop that specializes in "historical games," you found it. *Chutes and Ladders*, a game that first appeared in 1943. Your granddaughter rips open the wrapping paper, and instead of having the adoring smile you anticipated, she looks at you with disappointment and says, "Grandma, where's the Super Mario Maker?"

Some think the preference for electronics over traditional board games signals the end of civilization, while others believe it is the dawn of a new way of life. According to researchers, the answer is actually somewhere in between.[12] Regardless of what you think, video games portend for life on the planet, and playing them can positively affect your cognition,[13] and ttherefore they are also a tool for preventing senior moments. Depending on the type of game, it can improve short-term memory,[14] reaction time,[15] and working memory.[16]

Central to the elevation of video games over non-electronic ones is that they enhance neuroplasticity, the ability of the brain to make new connections.[17] So which games are most beneficial?

Instead of me making particular recommendations or endorsing a product, look for specific features of a game, such as using strategies, decision-making, and problem-solving. And if you cannot make a choice, just ask your granddaughter what you should choose. I have found that children are often the best authorities in choosing video games that require the skills necessary for enhanced cognition.

Video games are helpful in creating activities that target the general components of cognition, each of which can help prevent senior moments.

Non-Electronic Games

While video games have surged in popularity, do not dismiss the power of non-electronic games. Probably the king of all non-electronic games is chess, where virtually every time a piece is moved, the six skills go into play.[18] Games exercise the brain in the way physical activity exercises the body. The more you play, the better the results. Some games focus on spotting differences, others stimulate recall, and still others enhance concentration.

Regardless of the type of games you're playing, improved memory functions will always be the result. Best of all, you'll be having fun on your own or with some friends while exercising your brain.

Games, especially those that involve complex moves like chess, bridge, etc., offer efficient and effective methods helping in the development of neurons. Play them daily.

Participate in Discussions

When was the last time you gathered with friends to talk about a pressing social issue, book, or a controversial topic, such as how

Michelangelo's study of anatomy affected every sculptor who followed him? Most likely, your gatherings are more social, less esoteric, and have no objective other than renewing or reinforcing friendships. Yet, discussions—the exchange of ideas—are socially and psychologically refreshing and can serve as a vehicle for cognitive growth.

One of the most exciting and challenging activities I was involved in was a writing group that met once a month where we discussed our individual projects. Throughout the two hours we met, each of Goodwin and Miller's skills was used. The positive effects of discussions also apply to online discussion groups.[19] Book clubs are natural venues for creating the benefits of discussions. Regardless of whether they are open-ended (give us a review of the book) or topic-driven (what was the hero's journey?), they are good for the brain's health.

Get involved in a regular discussion group, in person or online, and routinely contribute to the conversation.

Purposefully Get Lost

You may wonder why I am suggesting you do something so bizarre as getting lost on purpose. Think of it as a dress rehearsal for physical and psychological feelings you might have when abandoned by Siri, as I was in the backroads of North Carolina. I had been relying on my GPS to get me from the airport in Charlotte to Boone. As I turned onto a dirt road what was supposed to be "Addison Lane," I saw a large sign that read:

REGARDLESS OF WHAT SIRI SAYS

YOU ARE NOT AT 5428 ADDISON ROAD

THIS IS PRIVATE PROPERTY. SHOO!

Without the comfort of having Siri calmly tell me where to go, or friendly locals pointing me in the right direction, I was forced to find my way using logic and memory. We have become so dependent upon technology that when it fails, we often are at a loss for what to do.

I am not suggesting you go to the most dangerous part of town and blindly walk through it at midnight. Select a safe area and venture during daylight hours either by car or on foot for a block or two. When you begin feeling slightly lost, stop and start mapping out either on paper or aurally (paper is better) how to get home. This rehearsal activity does two things. The first is allowing you to experience the emotion of being lost so you can try the disorientation strategies while in a structured and safe setting so when you are lost for real, you will be less anxious.[20] The second is requiring you to use the six skills in order to get home.

Getting lost on purpose will prepare you physically and psychologically for disorientation. Additionally, you will have a more controlled setting for trying out strategies and methods.

Create "What If" Scenarios

The military is adept at creating "war games," a misnomer that downplays the importance of the activity.[21] In war simulations, alternative scenarios are created that cover all eventualities. Sometimes that involves deciding what a military planner would do if either "a" or "b" occurred. For example, what should the United States do if Putin chooses a) not to use tactical nuclear weapons or b) to use them? Decision trees lead to endless "what if" scenarios that send planners to the next "what if" level. It is much like what you faced when your grandchild asked, "Why is the sky blue, Grandpa?" Regardless of your response, it probably will be followed by more "why" questions until your only answer is, "I don't know" or "Go out and play."

In your mind, create a decision tree where you are required to think about eventualities. When you have made a decision, ask yourself again, "but, what if," continually posing the question until you have exhausted all possibilities. Increasing the time you spend on active activities may not directly prevent senior moments, but it creates a background more conducive to preventing them.

CHAPTER 8

Fortifying and Retrieving Memories

The wisest man I ever knew taught me something I never forgot. And although I never forgot it, I never quite memorized it either. So what I'm left with is the memory of having learned something very wise that I can't quite remember.

—GEORGE CARLIN[1]

GEORGE CARLIN'S QUIRKY QUOTE HIGHLIGHTS THE TWO SIDES of memories: their creation and retrieval. If we understand the dynamics of their creation, we can fortify events so they will be more easily retrieved. For example, attending to someone who is giving you directions that will be important for you getting to a destination. There are situations where it is not sufficient just to create feature-rich memories, but also you might need methods for encouraging their retrieval. In the above example, you may have created wonderful visualizations of the route. However, that might not be enough for you to remember how many left turns you will need to make before turning right. A specific retrieval method might be necessary.

CREATING MEMORIES

For some memories many of the critical elements for creating a feature-rich memory are in place. Such is the case with my memory of a motorcycle trip I took in 1965 with a friend in the middle of the night from Pittsburgh to Greenwich Village. Even though it happened more than fifty years ago, I can describe the trip as if it happened yesterday. But other memories—ones that are feature-poor—we often cannot remember regardless of the number and type of retrieval aids used. So, how are memories created?

Let's do a simple, quick test. Briefly list any three methods you can recall that I described in any of the previous chapters. Take your time, and don't look back at the chapters! Now, what was it about each of them that facilitated retrieval? Most likely, the methods you remembered were associated with something concrete and or visual. For example, I used helping my father make sausages to show how various types of senior moments are similar yet distinct. I told the story of the Abbess comparing life to a glass of beer to emphasize the need to eliminate myths. And I compared a sleek Tesla with an ill-fated Edsel traveling to the same city to exemplify that various approaches can be used to solve the same problem. Each of these stories creates memories with visual retrieval hooks.[2] Each of the above stories is feature rich.

Feature-poor memories consist primarily of words. Here is an example from earlier in the book: "Procrastination is often seen as a major reason seniors do not complete tasks. However, what may appear to be procrastination may be your inability to multitask." Now, there is nothing wrong with these two sentences (if there were, I would not have included them in the book), but to retrieve this thought a week after you read it, you would be relying on your ability to retrieve abstractions—the words. Contrast the above with the following sentences: That roof repair you were to complete before the rainy season is now a funnel with water dripping directly onto your bed. The garden, which at one time was your pride and joy, is overgrown with weeds that are sucking the life out of your daffodils. As your project list grew, so did the number of unfinished "to-do" activities.

Which excerpt do you think is easier to remember? The first feature-poor memory or the second feature-rich memory? The richness of a memory, and therefore the ease of its retrieval, is determined when it was created. While you cannot do anything to improve memories after their creation, you can enrich them by (1) **using multisensory aides**, (2) **creating connections**, and (3) **using repetitive vocalization**.

Using Multisensory Aides

Doug Jones, in *Bending Toward Justice: The Birmingham Church Bombing that Changed the Course of Civil Rights*, poignantly describes in 384 pages the events leading up to the bombing of the Sixteenth Street Baptist Church in Montgomery, Alabama.[3] As compelling as the book was, it does not have the impact of *Anti-Mass*, a sculpture created by Cornelia Parker and exhibited at the DeYoung Museum in San Francisco.

Parker hung eight hundred pieces of charred wood from the remnants of a Southern Black Baptist church destroyed by arson. As you enter the room where the sculpture is displayed, a burnt odor is pervasive, and for me, seeing the charred wood evokes fifty-year-old memories of my involvement in the civil rights movement. The memory I recalled when standing in front of the sculpture was more vivid than any retrieved by words.

Feature-rich configurations, like *Anti-Mass*, which is infused with two modalities, sight and smell, excite more parts of the brain than feature-poor configurations and as a result, are easier to retrieve.[4] The easier a memory can be retrieved, the less likely senior moments related to memory will occur. Six years after seeing *Anti-Mass*, the memory of what I first saw and smelled remains strong.

When creating a memory that you know will need to be retrieved at a later date, involve as many modalities as possible.

Creating Connections

Think of connections as a spider's web, touching just one strand will evoke movement throughout the web, alerting the spider that lunch is being served. A similar sequence begins when I listen to the Beach Boys hit *409*. The song acts like the insect that lands in the spider's web; it lights up connections in my brain: I'm back in Allentown, Pennsylvania, in 1963 on a Saturday night cruising with my best friends and wondering how we can get someone to buy us a six-pack of Horelocker's Beer.

The connections my brain made in 1963 when it was storing the experience still exist. The presence of any of those elements can trigger a sixty-year-old memory of a formative part of my life. Memories with abundant connections are easier to retrieve than ones with few. Think of easily retrieved memories as three-dimensional pictures with sounds, odors, and textures the brain has broken apart and stored in pieces, ready to be reassembled when any of the connections to the experience appear.[5] The more connections, the higher the probability the brain can retrieve the memory.[6]

Using Repetitive Vocalization

You just asked a stranger if they could direct you to an address only a few blocks away that Siri will not recognize. Unfortunately, the stranger's directions involve four turns, and you do not have paper and a pencil to write them down. What do you do? Either vocally or sub-vocally, try to repeat all of the words. The method will usually work—getting you to the destination or close to it. Years ago, before personal GPS was available, I was trying to meet a friend at a rental car return in the Charlotte airport. I was notorious for having a poor sense of direction, and the maze of under- and overpasses made me feel I had just entered a world designed by someone with schizophrenia. Despite vocalizing the seven-part direction, I never got it correct, and what should have been a ten-minute drive ended up being a one-hour torturous journey.

Repetitive vocalization can be effective if what you are committing to memory is simple and short.[7] For example, repeating a phone number until you can enter it into your cell phone or write it down is fine. The reason repetition works may be analogous to how a wall's color becomes more vivid with each layer of paint. However, using this method with anything more complicated— like multiple-turn driving instructions—will most likely result in a memory riddled with errors.

Use vocalized repetition to remember a limited number of things for a short period.

RETRIEVING MEMORIES

As rich as your memories may have been at their creation, for various reasons their strength may have faded over time. You may not have had enough sleep, you may need to retrieve the memory in a noisy environment, your mind is full of worries, etc. Regardless of the reason, your frazzled brain needs a bit of help. Assistance comes in the form of **(1) cues and tags, (2) lists, and (3) numbers**.

Cues and Tags

During my younger days, I always had unique cars. My first car was a Goliath, a car made by the Borgward Company in Germany that went bankrupt and sold its equipment to a company in Mexico that made washing machines. My second car was a sleek Alfa Romeo that I needed a screwdriver to start, and a third was a Volkswagen painted "banana yellow" for $49 that my immigrant

Jewish mother refused to enter. As I got older and cars became increasingly similar, what I drove started looking like many others on the road. And as I became even older and less observant of where I parked my car, my white Acura SUV, from a distance, looked like scores of others in the Costco parking lot. On one occasion, I wheeled my cart for twenty minutes back and forth in an area the size of three football fields, looking for my car. I am sure I appeared to be a demented homeless man needing psychiatric help.

Since I knew I could not find a car unique enough to avoid another embarrassing situation, I decided to use something that would help me locate it—an iridescent small soccer ball held high by a rod that could be spotted anywhere in a parking lot. When people asked if I was a soccer coach or a player, I explained that it was a cue for my increasingly addled mind. Now, when entering the Costco parking lot, I see other cars with similar balls waving to their owners whose memory might be worse than mine.

The importance of cues goes beyond their comedic value in Costco's parking lot: They can be a quality-of-life strategy. A senior with mild dementia living alone could not remember how to turn on the heater in her apartment. Instead of explaining the steps orally, I taped pictures on the wall above her thermostat. One was a woman shivering, and underneath the picture was an arrow pointing right, indicating the direction the thermostat dial should be moved when she was cold. Next to that picture was another one of a woman sweating profusely with an arrow pointing left. My patient could raise or lower the heat when no one was present by following the sequence.

Cues and tags act as triggers when your ability to remember has deteriorated.

Lists

For our entire lives, we have relied upon "internal" lists. Our partner sends us to the store to buy milk, bread, and salami. A coworker asks you to send him four different documents. Usually, you rely on your memory for these and countless other tasks. However, as we age, items on our internal lists mysteriously disappear or are inexplicably replaced by other unintended objects.

I was not immune from this. A few years ago, I started having problems remembering which items in my pantry needed restocking. I have over seventy-five jars filled with assorted beans, spices, grains, etc. To compose my weekly marketing list accurately, I would need to go through everything and determine which items needed restocking. It was an unwelcome task. After all, how difficult should it be to remember five or six things? As a result, I would come back from the supermarket with duplicates of items in ample supply and forget ones needed for the evening meal—a senior moment evident when I looked at an empty garlic powder container next to four jars of turmeric. I eliminated my pantry senior moments by putting a removable red sticker on each jar as its contents became low. I also use different symbols to identify the types of food (e.g., gains, beans, seeds, etc.).

> *Cues and tags can be used as "training wheels" within strategies designed to improve memory, or they can become an acceptable part of your daily activity that endures.*

Numbers

In the past, when I left my house, I often forgot one or more items, such as my keys, cell phone, or wallet. My senior moment of forgetting vital objects ceased when I said the following mantra as I left my house. "I must have three things before I leave." Even more compelling was pasting the number "3" on the door.

When you use a number as a memory tool (e.g., three objects needed before leaving the house), the number becomes an effective magical recall device.[8] By relying on a number to remind you of things that are needed, the likelihood of forgetting them is drastically reduced. The use of numbers may not have as significant an effect on retrieval as vivid images, but it is an easy method for preventing many senior moments.

Using numbers to represent items to be remembered or tasks to be performed is a simple, effective method for enhancing memory. However, it is more appropriate for a limited number of items than for a large amount.

Chapter 9

Focus

Whenever you want to achieve something, keep your eyes open, concentrate and make sure you know exactly what it is you want. No one can hit their target with their eyes closed.

—Paulo Coelho[1]

Brazilian novelist Paulo Coelho got it half right. When you are learning something you want to execute with perfection, focus intently. Focus as if nothing else in the world matters. But when you achieve your goal, close your eyes and become the Zen archer who needs neither thoughts nor vision to hit a bull's-eye.

Our brains are fickle organs, constantly acting more like a hyperactive child than the most complicated entity in the universe. How can something with so much power become distracted from calculating numbers in a loan package by the sound of the tinkling bell on a child's bicycle? Should it not realize that putting together a document that could change your life is more important than wondering which neighborhood child is making so much noise? Unfortunately, noise trumps logic.

Distractibility, a cause of many senior moments, has its origins deep in our genetic history.[2] If our ancestors were engrossed in admiring a flower, they might not have heard the faint sounds of something lurking in the forest. If they continued to focus on the beauty of a new bud, they might become a velociraptor's dinner. Today, we do not have to worry about becoming a dinosaur's meal, yet the brain stubbornly refuses to give up distractibility. Maybe it believes the next dinosaur age will be next week? And when that happens, you will be thanking the brain for saving your life and, therefore, its life. It makes no difference to the brain that what was a survival skill fifty thousand years ago is now unnecessary. Since we cannot wait a million years for our brains to realize dinosaurs no longer exist, we need to find another way of bridling our genetic preferences. We can do it by (1) **monitoring**, (2) **incubating mindfulness, and (3) reducing stress.**

MONITORING

Think of monitoring as a parent watching over a child who constantly needs guidance. Knowing that his mother "has eyes in the back of her head" is enough to prevent some behaviors. Unfortunately, as soon as his mother leaves, he is back playing with the electrical outlet. In study after study, it became clear to researchers that just being aware of an undesirable behavior can reduce its occurrence.[3] This may not be a way of permanently preventing a senior moment, but it is effective in reducing the occurrences. You can (1) **monitor speech acts** or (2) **monitor physical behaviors.**

Monitoring Speech Acts

In the wonderful 1957 movie *The Last Hurrah*, Spencer Tracy's political sidekick repeats everything so often that everyone affectionally calls him "Ditto." Terms less endearing were used to describe a man I knew who repeated stories at almost every social gathering. While some friends patiently waited for the punchline, which they could recite verbatim, others began wondering if this was the first sign of dementia—which it was not. I suggested that during the next party, he use a counter that recorded every story he told. All he had to do was depress the clicker whenever he told a story, and it did not make any difference if he thought it was one he had never told or one familiar to most people. Just click it. According to his partner, the number of repeated stories dramatically declined. Just monitoring—becoming more aware—was sufficient to lower it.

Identify a speech behavior you want to change, and note it electronically, manually, or with the help of someone. Augment this method with others designed to directly reduce the senior moment.

Monitoring Physical Behaviors

From inside his house, a man would often go to the window facing the street and peer out. It was a behavior that occurred not only when he was alone but also with friends who often joked that he was patrolling for terrorists. He was not aware how often the behavior occurred. Still, after reoccurring jokes about his stalking, he decided to address the problem and used the same type of counter my other client did to monitor his stories. The result? Fewer visits to the window. Counting behaviors is easier than counting speech acts. Speech acts are ephemeral; behaviors are more visual, lasting, and easier to monitor.

Counting the occurrence of a behavior increases awareness, sometimes the only thing necessary for preventing senior moments, but usually, the method should be augmented by others having a more direct influence.

INCUBATING MINDFULNESS

Think of the brain as if it is a twelve-inch apple pie. As you drive on a busy highway, your brain says, "I need ten inches of concentration to keep you safe." That gives it only two inches for unimportant activities such as reading advertisements along the highway. Your admiration for the flashing billboard evaporates when you realize you just passed your exit and will not be able to turn around for fifteen miles. Your friends in the car just shake their heads and mumble to each other about your atrocious senior driving skills.

It would be great if you could put the brain into overdrive and recruit a few more million neurons to handle the additional demands of reading the latest eye-catching billboard while still driving safely—but that is not how your brain works. Instead of recruiting some unused cells assigned for walking (you do not need them since you are sitting), it pulls a few inches of the pie away from the ten inches required for safe driving.[4] The result? The more attention you pay to the signs, the fewer inches you have available for realizing a semi-truck is bearing down on you. By ignoring your brain's limitations, you set in motion the conditions for creating a senior moment and possibly a tragic accident.

Although you cannot stretch twelve inches of concentration into fifteen inches, you can use mindfulness methods that will enable you to focus your attention on a specific activity while keeping distractions to a minimum. The term "mindfulness" is one of those words whose meaning changes with whoever uses it. I have found the one used by Jon Kabat-Zinn to be the simplest and most practical. *Mindfulness is awareness that arises through paying attention, on purpose, in the present moment, nonjudgmentally.*[5] As straightforward as Kabat-Zinn's definition is, mindfulness for a person who has been meditating for twenty years is not the same as it is for a single mom who works eight hours a day, has children who need attention, and is dealing with argumentative relatives.

Mindfulness involves looking at your world without filters. This concept of the "naïve observer" is a foundational idea for the school of philosophy known as phenomenology.[6] Simply put, its adherents suggest initially observing before labeling. For example, instead of having an initial reaction that the person you see on the street is rich, in your mind, describe their well-tailored suit, shoes that you know cost more than your monthly mortgage payment, and the handbag that costs double that. This way of observing involves "bracketing" what you see before judging. The value of observation goes far beyond withholding judgments. It can become a handy tool for preventing senior moments related to inattention.

The psychological benefits of mindfulness or increased awareness have been well documented and have seeped into therapeutic approaches as alternatives to drug therapy and "talk" counseling.[7] You can become more mindful by **(1) prioritizing, (2) taking breaks, and (3) switching activities**.

Prioritizing

On your desk are unpaid bills, receipts for an Amazon order that disappeared from your porch, a shirt that cannot be worn until you sew on a button, and a grocery list for tonight's dinner. Where do you begin? Often the selection is random and can lead to embarrassing events. Have you ever been faced with many things to do, and you do not know where to start? Prioritization is a nontechnical skill critical in many areas, yet its importance in preventing senior moments is often overlooked.[8]

There are various ways of prioritizing activities ranging from difficulty in execution to available time. Any of them will help you focus, as it did for a man who usually had at least five household tasks he was required to do every day and never seemed to finish any. One of them, cleaning the kitchen, would routinely take a long time. When it was especially filthy, he would not have enough time to complete his other responsibilities. A simple solution he used was to start with the activities that required the least amount of time and work his way through others until the only task left was cleaning the kitchen.

Another way to tackle responsibilities is to prioritize them based on how easy they are to complete. For example, a woman was experiencing disorientation while driving in familiar areas. Her approach to reducing her anxiety was repeatedly driving in the neighborhood, hoping that her discomfort would continue to fade with each visit. Unfortunately, experiencing multiple failures did not reduce her anxiety. Instead, it reinforced her negative self-image and codified disorientation into something unchangeable. That view stopped when instead of just driving through the neighborhood, she ventured into only the first block and was able to retreat before "getting lost," and developing anxiety. For many people, especially those with a history of failures, the ease of completion may be the most appropriate priority.[9]

Sometimes, however, you must do a task, not because it is easy or enjoyable, but because it is required if you want to avoid negative consequences. While doing something out of necessity is a method of prioritizing tasks, it is most likely one of the least enjoyable ways to get things done.

Taking Breaks

When I was much younger, I could sit at the computer and write for hours, only taking breaks for coffee and the bathroom. But as I got older, I realized that lengthy sessions, while producing many pages, resulted in a product that was not what it had been in past years. The senior moments resulting from marathon writing sessions were more than embarrassing—they resulted in article rejections. The method I developed to prevent writing senior moments was to limit the amount of time without taking a break to one hour, followed by a fifteen-minute break. During the break, I took care of bathroom needs, ate a snack, made coffee, and sometimes used the time for mild exercise (e.g., jumping rope). When you have established guidelines for your breaks, adjust them based on the level of concentration the activity requires, how alert or exhausted you feel that day, and the total time you have for a distraction.

There is no magic number of break minutes you should adopt. Start with a short amount of time that will not disrupt your activity, then gradually increase the number of minutes until the next scheduled break. A good start is a 4:1 ratio (e.g., for every sixty minutes of work, impose a fifteen-minute break.

Switching Activities

The switching activities method is similar to the taking a break method, except that you stop doing one type of activity and immediately start another. The simple act of switching frees up the brain to focus better when the first activity is resumed.[10] For example, switching from a purely cognitive activity like writing to something physical like running refreshes the brain.[11] This increases focus and decreases the odds of a senior moment. One experiment that examined the effect walking had on thinking found that walking was effective in increasing the accuracy of tasks that involved cognition. [12]

Switching from a cognitive to a physical activity provides a "refreshment" period that results in improved cognitive performance.

REDUCING STRESS

How often have you experienced so much stress you felt like running away or doing something awful to the person causing it? When you are stressed, the brain is flooded with hormones intended for short-term emergencies. Remaining in a stressful condition over a long period of time can kill brain cells.[13] And even if the stress is short-term, it reduces the brain's ability to process and use information accurately.

As much as you want to interact with your grandkids following a horrendous argument with a friend, you cannot. Stress is forcing your brain to prioritize attention from the present to the argument.[14] Your granddaughter asks you a simple question about dinner, and you respond by saying, "We'll watch cartoons later." She is confused, and your daughter wonders if you should be trusted to watch the grandkids by yourself. Although stress may not directly lead to senior moments, it does set up the brain for creating conditions conducive to a senior moment. We seriously understate the destructive nature of stress on the brain.

You can reduce stress by **(1) choosing appropriate goals, (2) completing tasks, and (3) meditating**.

Choosing Appropriate Goals

Inappropriate goals can result in stress. For example, a person who suffered a stroke that left him with permanent weakness in his right arm and leg decided that his first goal in recovery would be to play tennis once again, an activity he loved and had done for more than fifty years. Given his level of disability, being able to play tennis—even just volleying—was going to be unreachable. Stress was created for this gentleman not only when he got onto the court, but even thinking about it.

> *Judiciously choose your goal. It is more important to be successful with a simple, easily achieved goal than failing because you chose an inappropriate goal.*

Completing Tasks

What you may not realize is that the consequences of procrastinating can produce stress, which can result in physical problems, cause emotional instability, and lead to problems in cognitive functioning.[15] Difficulties in any of these areas can result in senior moments.

The more tasks you leave unfinished, the greater the stress you create. Complete a specific number of tasks before starting any new ones.

Meditating

When meditation is mentioned, one might think of a robe-clad monk sitting in a cave contemplating nothing, or a Hare Krishna follower from your college days accosting you at an airport. However, meditation is not necessarily tied to a religion or an airport postulate. Meditation is a millennium-old technique that has been given scientific credence in recent years as a neurological tool for calming the mind and focusing attention.[16] I heard a young monk startle his audience—including me—by saying, "Meditation is nothing more than a psychological trick that cleans the mind." Recent research on the benefits of meditation confirms the monk's folksy thoughts.[17]

Meditation can involve thinking about nothing—a concept difficult to grasp by many people—or focusing on one thing. Many new meditators find it difficult to focus on "nothing" or "emptiness." A more accessible approach is to focus on one object, such as a flickering candle, a simple mantra (repeated words or phrases), and the inhalation and exhalation of breath, to mention just a few. You can meditate while sitting, walking, or working. Many years ago at a retreat, a monk assigned me the job of weeding a garden for one hour. After only a few minutes, I could only think about weed removal. The result was an increased awareness of everything I did for the next few hours. The purpose of meditation—regardless of the activity—is to allow the brain to "clear" and, by so doing, refresh itself, as one does in a cold shower on a hot day.

Most conventional meditation approaches are effective. It is less important to find the best and more essential to choose one that is easy to use. If any form of meditation seems too daunting, focus on a single everyday activity, like washing dishes for ten minutes. Concentrate on every movement you make, from turning on the water to putting the dish back into the cabinets. Sometimes I choose to meditate while sitting. At other times, my meditation involves concentrating on each note I play on my flute. As the young monk said, meditation is a psychological trick. Be less concerned with its form and more with the outcome.

I have found that meditating first thing in the morning and just before I go to bed has the most significant effects on "clearing out the daily garbage." My morning meditation slows me down for the day, and my evening meditation results in better sleep. Start with ten minutes per session and gradually increase your time to twenty minutes. After a few weeks of consistent practice, you should experience increased clarity in your observations, thinking, and sleep. Increasing awareness of thoughts, actions, and behaviors significantly raises your consciousness and reduces the possibility of senior moments.

There is no right or wrong way of meditating. The purpose of meditating is to clear out the clutter that impedes the mind's ability to focus. Find one that you like and is effective.

Chapter 10

Managing Your Environment

"Incredible change happens in your life when you decide to take control of what you do have power over instead of craving control over what you don't."

—Steve Maraboli[1]

Steve Maraboli's take on the importance of focusing on what you can control rather than what you cannot is important for structuring an environment that makes it more difficult for senior moments to develop. It was a lesson put into practice by a manager of a major corporation who believed his senior moments were spinning out of control.

At work, department meetings were becoming increasingly hostile, with two factions fighting to control company policy. As the stress level of the meetings increased, the manager's ability to focus and offer clear reasons for his positions suffered. The group that opposed his policy suggestions viewed his verbal stumbling as a signal that his cognitive powers were declining. "After all, the guy is nearing retirement," he heard one of them say. There was little he could do to change the view that age was synonymous with an addled brain, so he took a different approach. Before every meeting, he brought breakfast goods for everyone to share. His opposition still believed his policies were wrong, but a simple act of kindness lowered the verbal hostility and his stress level.

Think of structure as a framework for action. In the military, a rigid command and control network assures orders given by a Pentagon general are followed by soldiers stationed in the most remote outpost in the far east. The reliance on structure can be found in hospitals' strict adherence to surgical procedures, like accounting for the number of sponges used before an incision is closed. When structure is ignored, forgotten, or defective, the brain will struggle to work through the chaos. Unfortunately, there is just so much it can do.[2] There are three methods that can be used to manage your environment: **(1) create structure, (2) reduce interfering variables, and (3) restrict incoming data.**

CREATE STRUCTURE

Think of pictures you have seen of a hurricane's aftermath. Houses still standing often have critical parts missing, such as a roof, windows, etc. Although it is filled with "holes," you can still tell it was a house. This is analogous to an impaired memory process: the gist of the memory is still present despite missing parts.[3]

At seventy-seven, I take comfort in my morning routine of making coffee at 4:00 a.m., meditating for twenty minutes, reading and responding to emails, and finally, a short run with my dog. Even though I do not have dementia, if the sequence is disrupted—or God forbid, I cannot do any of the activities—I become irritable. You can recreate structure by **(1) making internal rules external, (2) creating stations, (3) replicating stable settings, (4) reducing clutter, (5) thinking linearly, and (6) simplifying.**

MAKING INTERNAL RULES EXTERNAL

External rules can replace lost or defective internal ones.[4] For example, a client who had been a professional chef before retiring began having memory problems. Prior to the problem's onset, he cooked the signature dish of his restaurant so many times that he performed each of the steps automatically. But as his memory problems progressed, in the chaos of a busy kitchen he would forget where he was in a cooking sequence. The result was that essential ingredients were sometimes missing or doubled. He solved his problem by posting a note above his cook station that listed each step for a complicated dish. For example, for one dish, he listed the following steps:

1. Prep items

2. Sauté vegetables

3. Braise meat

4. Sauce ingredients

5. Plate

6. Inspect

7. Signal waiter

Making internal rules external can be as easy as using a note as the chef did or setting up a process like the one I use for remembering to alternate running shoes; placing the shoes I used today behind the ones I will use tomorrow.

> *Although we rely on our memory for structure, when memory begins to fail, structure should be externalized to avoid senior moments.*

CREATING STATIONS

For years I used the same area for writing as I did for tying flies, believing that the convenience of having both activities in the same area outweighed the time necessary to find feathers within piles of manuscript papers. The outcome? Documents, such as the manuscript for this book, became mixed in with hooks and thread needed to tie a Micky Finn. A lack of structure led to flies missing items necessary for fooling fish and essays on social responsibility ending with descriptions of how to fish a Lefty's Deceiver. Now I keep everything related to writing in one area of my office and everything associated with fly-tying in another.

Let us say that when you leave your house every morning, you randomly place your cell phone, keys, and wallet into whatever pockets are available, or you just dump everything into your purse. Halfway to work, you panic wondering if the cell phone you need for an important call is still at home and if you have money to pay for the bridge toll. By physically separating objects or activities, the brain will mirror the same maneuver.[5]

How often have you put something in one place, knowing you will need to move it eventually? Maybe you placed a piece of paper on a pile that is only a waystation for placement somewhere else. By consistently placing that cell phone in a specific pocket or area in your purse, the behavior begins the path toward automaticity. With each new consistent placement, the memory of where each item is should get stronger. How long will it take for you to automatically place a wallet into its designated pocket? Research says habits require between 18 and 254 days to form if consistently practiced.[6] It took me a month of placing my wallet seven days a week into my right front pocket before that behavior became automatic. When I leave my house, a comforting feeling develops when I feel my wallet in my right front pocket. Conversely, if I place it in any other pocket or forget it, I know something is wrong by the time I open the door. To make behaviors automatic, don't worry about how long it will take. Just remember the following two principles:

1. The longer you do a behavior, the more likely it will become automatic.

2. The more consistently you practice a behavior, the more likely it will become automatic.

Consistently place items in their designated place to create behaviors that are automatic. When the behavior becomes automatic, any deviation will signal you that something is wrong.

REPLICATING STABLE SETTINGS

You never forget your morning medications at home, but you forget to take them on vacation. Your partner would think this was humorous if it did not pose the possibility of endangering your heart by neglecting to take your blood thinner. You can spend your time pondering why you have difficulty remembering them on vacation but never at home, or you can do something less psychotherapeutic that takes less time and is more effective—replicate at your vacation location the most important features for pill taking at home. You do this by identifying the salient home features and duplicating them on vacation. For example, at home, pills are always in a daily pill box placed on the nightstand, a glass of water is next to the pillbox, and you eat breakfast only after you take the pills. Replicating these salient features will make it easier for your brain to recognize these as triggers for taking pills at a hotel in Tahiti.[7]

If you are able to avoid doing a specific senior moment in one setting but not others, replicate the most salient features of the successful setting. The more similar the settings, the less likely a senior moment will occur.

REDUCING CLUTTER

A client's office looked like a depository for whatever he no longer found necessary but with which he was unwilling to part. His desk was covered with papers that needed filing, pictures of a trip to Bermuda he took three years ago, and remnants of last night's dinner. A hoarder for many years, his office looked more like a neighborhood yard sale than the site of a successful real estate management company.

Clutter can be external or internal. Regardless of where it originates, it plays havoc with the brain's ability to function efficiently.[8] Remember the brain's ancestral tendency to direct attention to noise? Clutter may be just as much a distraction as noise and just as likely to cause senior moments. Although we do not know precisely how clutter affects the brain, we can witness its effects.[9] For example, when my client began having difficulty understanding conversations, his employees thought he was becoming senile, when in fact, during discussions in his office, objects scattered around the room triggered memories, distracting him.

The more your brain uses its energy to make sense of clutter, the less it will have to process new information.[10] Various explanations have been given for why hoarding occurs, ranging from psychological to physiological.[11] Regardless of the cause or the severity, keeping more than what is necessary increases the possibility of having senior moments at any stage of information processing. Clutter is more than annoying.

While external clutter is easy to handle, internal clutter proves more difficult. For example, a seventy-year-old woman I served in hospice would retell a story about being rejected when she was a twenty-year-old student teacher every time I came to visit. Sometimes she told the story as a stand-alone event, and other times she wove it into the conversation to make a point on an unrelated topic. The event was so traumatic that it vividly remained in her memory for over fifty years.

Clutter, whether internal or external, will reduce your ability to focus. Getting rid of external clutter may be as simple as putting objects back where they belong or just throwing away useless items. Internal clutter—those events you have struggled to overcome will be more difficult to eliminate but are just as disruptive or even more so than external clutter.

THINKING LINEARLY

Tibetans have a saying, "When you sit, sit. When you stand, stand, but whatever you do, don't wobble." While people tout multitasking as an efficient way for younger folks to work, the practice can lead to senior moments for older people.[12] A client found her weekly office meeting boring and a waste of time. Since her supervisor discussed so little of importance, she believed the best use of her time was to fill out paperwork as he spoke. She realized she could not "chew gum and walk" when instead of writing down an important date a contract was due, she was filling out her timesheet, missed the deadline, and was fired.

When you try to multitask, the brain divides its analytical power, making it more challenging to do even one correctly.[13] Multitasking does have its place when:

1. One task is physical, and the other cognitive (i.e., jogging while listening to music)

2. Doing something cognitive while waiting for a physical event to finish (i.e., writing a marketing list while waiting for eggs to boil)

3. Doing two cognitive tasks but separately (i.e., listening to the news, pausing it when you respond to emails, and repeating the process)

Einstein reportedly said, "Any man who can drive safely while kissing a pretty girl is simply not giving the kiss the attention it deserves."[14] Remember his pithy observation the next time you try to balance your checkbook while watching TV.

> *Do not multitask if you can avoid it. If you cannot, then only one task should involve cognition (e.g., listening to a conversation on television) and the other physical (e.g., putting away the dishes.)*

Simplifying

There is a story about the Buddha sitting in the woods with his disciples when a farmer frantically runs up to them and asks if anyone has seen his cows stampeding through the forest. The Buddha asked how many, and the farmer responded, "six." The farmer complained about all the work he had done to feed the cows, care for them, etc. He also lamented how the loss of his cows shattered his plans for the future. After he left, the Buddha turned to his impoverished disciples and said, "Look how lucky you are. Since you do not have cows, you do not suffer as that farmer does."

Life continues to grow more complicated, a trend accelerated by our reliance on technology. Mind you, I still prefer using my Word program rather than a yellow legal pad. Still, our dependence on technology has an unintentional consequence—it denies the brain a chance to problem solve. We once relied on maps to prevent getting lost while driving. Now we are so dependent on GPS that your grandchildren may ask, "Grandma, what's a map?" While GPS is a great advancement for drivers like me who constantly get lost even with a map, it can create a panic situation when your GPS freezes or you enter the hinterlands and read "no signal." The more complicated our lives, the greater opportunity for senior moments to occur. Take, for example, refrigerators.

Until recently, they served only two purposes: to keep food cold or frozen. Now, you can buy a refrigerator that notifies you when food is expired, live-streams its contents to you through your cell phone, checks your grocery list, streams music or TV on its front panel, keeps track of the whole family's schedules, sends reminders, asks daily trivia questions, orders deliveries, responds to voice commands, and makes over eight pounds of ice a day—all while keeping food cold or frozen.

Think about all of the refrigerator's circuits and connections that need to function perfectly for this contraption to work beyond the manufacturer's warranty period. A slight microburst of energy, a faulty connection, or a bump when your grandchild pretends she is racing at Daytona, and what follows is an acrimonious discussion with the customer service representative with an accent you cannot understand.

Simplifying things will reduce the possibility of having a senior moment. Simplification can be physical (e.g., doing fewer activities) or cognitive (e.g., limiting the number of recipes you try to create.)

Reduce Interfering Variables

We think of noise as sounds that can interfere with hearing. However, when preventing senior moments, noise is anything that either masks sound to which the brain is trying to attend or draws attention away from it. The jackhammer outside your window might make it impossible to hear what your partner is saying (masking). But your distraction could be just as great if your mind shifts its attention to the sound of a child dribbling a basketball while you sit in the park reading this book.

In psychology and the visual arts, there is a concept known as "figure-ground," which asserts that the brain is always on the lookout for anything distinct from its background.[15] Look at any painting from the Renaissance. You will see how the painters of the fourteenth to the sixteenth century were obsessed with this principle. They wanted to draw the viewer's attention to a specific object or person in their painting. The same phenomenon exists—the need to separate what is more important from what is less important—in how we perceive the world. It becomes a problem when the brain focuses on something you do not want to be the "figure," like the noise of a room air conditioner when you are trying to sleep in a motel room. Noise can be external as well as internal.

EXTERNAL NOISE

As a hospice volunteer, I was assigned to patients in nursing homes. At one facility, the staff was frustrated by their patient's lack of communication. They wanted to serve them but did not know how to enable their patients to discuss death. As I walked in the central hallway, I learned why the residents chose not to communicate; a cacophony of sounds came from each room. Imagine an environment with twenty televisions that were always on, tuned to different stations, and blaring at various volumes. Not exactly an environment conducive to talking about the end of one's life. The staff viewed the televisions as entertainment for the patients. While the televisions did serve that purpose, they also overloaded the patients' auditory systems. The simple solution? Lower the volume, turn off the TVs, or close the patients' doors.

The more you can limit external noise's muddling effects; the less likely a senior moment will occur. The impact of noise on your brain is similar to dust sneaking into an old-fashioned pocket watch with gears, escapements, jewels, posts, and what-nots. Introduce a speck of dust into the watch, and a gear freezes, spokes pull out of line, etc. The watch still operates but fluctuates hourly instead of providing accurate times. The effects of external noise on information processing are similar. You will not throw a brain gear when listening to a Grateful Dead CD, but you may not understand the article you are reading on finance with "Sugar Magnolia" playing in the background. The more you can reduce noise, the less likely senior moments related to listening will occur.

External noise can come from sight, smell, touch, or sound.[16] For example, you are looking at a serene scene, and enjoying it until a small animal moves in the distance. Without warning, your brain disregards the scenery and focuses on the hopping bunny. Listen to a Brahms concerto at the symphony, and with each cough from the audience, your brain diverts attention to the "noise." Your brain can't help itself, just like the brain of predator animals is programmed to act in specific biologically determined ways.[17] In humans, the behavior may be a leftover survival technique. That would explain how music can function as noise. For example, how often have you turned on music while reading, believing your comprehension would not suffer? It could have been Beethoven's "Moonlight Sonata" or The Beetle's "Let It Be." The effects of various music genres are controversial because variables such as mood, musical preference, and arousal make it challenging to assess their impact on comprehension.[18] If you have a history of few problems with a particular type of music, continue listening to it—just be sure you are not deceiving yourself about your ability to comprehend. If the music interferes, stop listening. If you believe you must have music in the background but know it impacts comprehension, reduce the volume.

What attracts human and animal brains in the environment is anything that stands out from the background. The brain will unexpectedly shift focus like a hyperactive child from something static (background) to what moves (figure). The more external noise present, the more it can impede precise information processing.[19] The less accurate information processing, the more likely a senior moment may occur. These intrusions (noise) can affect the comprehension of both spoken and written materials.[20]

When you have no control over the external noise (e.g., street construction), allow your brain time to adapt to the noise before you begin executing a behavior that in the past led to a senior moment.[21] For unknown reasons, the brain can move potentially distracting elements into the background.[22] When I was doing research that required a video camera in the room with a subject, I would not start recording until ten to fifteen minutes had passed. But sometimes, you cannot adapt to noise, such as when trying to follow a recipe. I have a rule when cooking and someone is in the kitchen talking to me. Whenever I need to read instructions or measure quantities, all conversation ceases. I created my "kitchen noise rule" when my conversation with guests while cooking resulted in an inedible main course at a Super Bowl party. The debacle is still a favorite senior moment story told by the party's guests about my kimchi pierogis.

External noise—even music—rarely helps with comprehension. Whenever possible, reduce or eliminate external noise. If that is not possible, give your brain a few minutes to adapt.

INTERNAL NOISE
Internal noise consists of thoughts or feelings that make it difficult to concentrate on the present. For example, you wonder how to pay next month's bills while a friend talks about her favorite television show. She asks you what you think, and your response— having nothing to do with the question—makes your friend wonder what is going on in your head. Many years ago, I attempted to determine how internal noises were successfully controlled by master clinicians—those acclaimed by their profession as "the best of the best."[23] These clinicians were known for their ability to stay focused on their client's needs regardless of where the conversation went. I interviewed five and asked how it was possible for them to remain focused for the entire fifty-minute session. One clinician said, "I park whatever problems I'm dealing with outside

the room, and the only thing that exists for me when I am with the client is their problem."

Other clinicians cited methods that "cleaned the mind" so they could focus. According to the clinicians, internal noise diverted their attention away from the present. I learned the importance of clearing internal noise when serving hospice patients. Conversations with dying people are more critical than "everyday chatter." Following a discussion about how the San Francisco Giants are doing in the pennant race is quite different from a conversation on the need to forgive. To prepare myself for discussions like the latter, I would spend twenty minutes playing single notes on my flute as a way of focusing my mind on the present before I entered a patient's room.

When we demand our internal noises to stop, the mind often does the reverse—it amplifies them. A more effective approach is to use indirect strategies, which include meditation, sleep, and physical activities.

Internal noise can be more challenging to control than external noise. Many different approaches can be used to quell internal noise. Use whatever works for you.

Restrict Incoming Data

Too much data can create an unmanageable situation that can lead to senior moments. Think of a stream before a massive downpour. As long as the volume of rain stays below a certain number of inches, the stream stays within its banks. But with a downpour—even for a short time—there is the chance of flooding. The brain acts the same way. You can restrict the amount of data coming into your brain by reducing the data's **(1) speed** or **(2)** volume.

REDUCING THE DATA'S SPEED

Two academics did not think highly of each other. Still, their disagreements were never voiced publicly until one day when Professor "A" was rushing to complete a paper he would be presenting at a conference. In an email conversation with a collogue, he eviscerated Professor "B," ending with a series of expletives I will not mention here. Unfortunately, in his haste to hit "send," just to his colleague, he hit "send to everyone," which included 2,400 academics on a list, including me and Professor "B."

How often have you sent or did something like hit "send" realizing immediately the mistake you made? Bill Clinton was known for taking at least a few seconds before answering difficult questions. Lawyers routinely instruct clients to take their time before answering during a deposition or trial. Even Amazon has an option when you return merchandise to indicate you ordered it by mistake. When I was a child, we had play options called "take it back," allowing us to reverse words or actions. Unfortunately, there are some situations where you do not have a "take it back" option. However, you can prevent many gaffs by slowing down the information you are asking your brain to tackle. They include simple methods such as counting to five before hitting the send key, re-reading instructions, pausing before answering, etc.

Taking your time to act or respond will give your brain a few more seconds to access what you have just asked it to do.

REDUCING THE DATA'S VOLUME

We live in a world that saturates us with data. I know if I do not look at my inbox for a day, I will be swamped with so many unanswered emails that I will spend the next few hours just weeding through them. Being saturated with data is not limited to receiving multiple offers for merchandise I would never consider buying. Instead of looking at San Francisco's beautiful architectural skyline as I enter the city, my vision is inundated with billboards advertising everything from the latest iPhone to companies wanting to deliver everything from sandwiches to cars to my door. Yes, data is essential. Data is good, but like Emperor Franz Joseph's response to Mozart, maybe we have too much of it. Do you need to watch the news four times a day? How many of those emails do you need to read before deleting them? If you reduce the flow of data, your brain will thank you for the bit of relief you give it.

Any method for reducing data flow will help avoid senior moments caused by data overload.

Chapter 11

Practice, Practice, Practice

An out-of-towner lost in New York City asks a local how to get to Carnegie Hall.
The answer? Practice.

It is an old joke, but it contains enormous wisdom. I learned its importance when I took a woodcarving class from a master Japanese carver who specialized in carving monks: sitting monks, standing monks, praying monks, walking monks. Some people might view his focus on carving only monks as an obsession, but for my *sensei* (teacher) it was a path for carving perfection. On the first day of class he politely told us that if we wanted to learn how to carve monks, we were in the right place.

"We carve monks, only monks here."

Our first assignment was to carve a simple design onto a piece of square wood. From a set of tools I took out one knife and etched the design into the wood. Then, I took another for widening the line, followed by one to increase the depth of the cut. As I was about to select a fourth one, the teacher stopped in front of me.

"No," he said holding up one finger. "Only one, until you know."

He reached into my set of thirty tools and chose the simplest knife, one I thought was worthless.

"This one, only this one," he said.

For six months I only used that knife, learning how to do every imaginable cut with it. Sometimes I wondered if I could use that simple tool to build a house. From my sensei, I came to learn, repetitive and simple practice over a long period of time was the only way to develop mastery. It took six months and hundreds of hours before I was allowed to move on to another knife. Practice, not only for my sensei, but for anyone wishing to prevent a senior moment is essential. You can fine-tune your practice by **(1) structuring it, (2) making the behaviors automatic, and (3) testing for automaticity**.

STRUCTURE

Structured practicing can increase the quantity and quality of behaviors, whether scooping a ground ball or remembering where you are in a sequence.[1] A client wanted to become a better golfer. The joke in her weekly foursome was that "Jill never saw a tree she didn't want to hit." It became Jill's defining senior moment. She found a golf instructor who understood that unstructured practice could be worse than no practice, so he devised a practice strategy that included three essential elements: **(1) where to practice, (2) when to practice, and (3) how to practice**.

Where to Practice

Have you ever worked on a behavior for several weeks in anticipation of performing it? It could have been a new golf swing for a tournament or a bidding strategy for the game of bridge. In my case, it was a short flute piece I composed for my friend's wedding. I practiced the piece for at least one hour every day starting two months before the wedding. Days before the event, my flute produced more correct notes than I thought possible, more than enough to prevent embarrassment in front of friends and family.

So, on the day of his wedding, I was ready. My ego soared, and I thought, *Stand down, Matt Malloy* (considered the best Irish flutist); *you are about to be replaced by Stan Goldberg!*

As I approached the stage, I felt invincible, but something did not feel right as I went behind the microphone and looked out at the audience. I panicked, a feeling I should not have had. After all, did I not play this piece hundreds of times flawlessly? The battle between correct and wrong notes unfolded. How was it possible, I wondered, that there could be so little carryover of my practice successes to the actual performance?

The answer contained a simple principle I should have followed: if practice is to be successful, the sessions should be as similar as possible to the performance situation. I did the opposite. At home, I practiced sitting down. At the wedding, I stood. At home, I practiced in a room by myself. At the wedding, I faced more than two hundred people. At home, there was only silence. At the wedding, glasses were constantly clinking, and service people were mumbling to each other. How well did I do? "Flubbing" would be an understatement to describe my performance. My embarrassment could have been avoided if I had replicated in practice what I would experience during the live performance.[2]

> *When you practice, make sure your practice setting has similar features to the setting in which you will be displaying your new non-senior-moment behavior.*

When to Practice

When we practice usually has more to do with convenience than the principles of practice. In the previous flute example, I practiced at 7:00 a.m. every day when everyone in my house was still asleep, and I was yet to be burdened by a host of daily responsibilities. The time was perfect for harnessing my best level of alertness, but the wedding was to be held at 6:00 p.m., when my energy was usually drained. I trained to deliver a performance at my "best" times, yet I had to deliver the performance at the time of day when I was usually exhausted. I should have taken a lesson from US professional football teams when they played in Mexico City at an altitude of 7,349 feet. They arrived a week before the game to adapt to playing at that altitude.

Unfortunately, we cannot always select our energy level for performance, nor can we take a week like the NFL players did to practice at an unfamiliar altitude. But do the best you can to create conditions that mirror as closely as possible where your behavior will be performed.

When you practice, select situations that are similar to the one in which the behavior will be performed. The closer the two, the more likely your target behavior will be proficiently performed.

What to Practice

There are many things you can choose to practice, ranging from specific parts of the new behavior you want to master to how the behavior will be performed. Take the example of my client who sometimes had problems comprehending fast speech. In the past, during her book club sessions, she found that when someone spoke fast, she had more difficulty than when their speech was slow. Knowing the personalities of her friends, she knew it would be impossible to get them to slow down enough for her comprehension to improve. Instead of asking them to slow their speech, she practiced understanding rapid speech—the rate at which the discussions always occurred. She practiced listening to speakers using various speech rates, starting with snippets of slow speakers on YouTube and ending with ones whose speech approximated or exceeded the rate of her friends' speech.

Regardless of what you choose to practice, it should be done by initially selecting a goal that will be easily achieved, then move on to something slightly closer to the target, eventually arriving at the speed or complexity of your target behavior.

How to Practice

Bob Bowman, Mark Phelps's Olympic coach, believed the "how" of practice might be the most crucial element in workouts. It has been reported that he kept Phelps in the pool as long as his strokes and bodily movement were perfect. He would immediately take Phelps out of the water whenever his form deviated, arguing that practicing something that was not perfect was worse than not practicing at all.[3] Practicing perfectly is key to understanding why some efforts can produce automaticity of the desired behavior while others reinforce undesired behaviors.

One purpose of practice is to create memories sufficiently strong that they become automatic—that your brain does not have to think very much when it retrieves a memory. The stronger the memory, the easier it will be to retrieve, whether it is the sequence needed to initiate a computer program or remember all your grandchildren's names. Research suggests that the reason practice results in a better recall is it increases the size of the hippocampus, the part of the brain believed to be responsible for storing memories.[4] With repeated practice, the size of the hippocampus increases, which may allow for a better retention of new behaviors that will replace ones leading to senior moments. Regardless of what is happening in the hippocampus, the more you practice a behavior, the more likely the behavior you are trying to master will become automatic. And the more automated, the more likely it will replace a senior moment.[5]

Practice only the most perfect version of the behavior you are trying to make automatic. Practicing errors will only reinforce the variables that make it difficult for the undesired behavior to be eliminated.

MAKING BEHAVIORS AUTOMATIC

There is a sequence of events that helps make behaviors automatic, whether a ballet move, remembering why you are in the kitchen, or listening more carefully to someone giving you instructions on the phone. They involve **(1) identifying the most salient features of the behavior you want to become automatic, (2) repetition, and (3) consistent practice**.

Identifying the Salient Features

When trying to make a behavior automatic, it is important that you identify the most salient features of the behavior. This does not mean you should strip away everything else, but rather highlight the most important things you want to become automatic. For example, a client used much of his free time in the morning looking for items he would need throughout the day. The problem, he realized, did not begin in the mornings but rather the day before when he would place items down when he no longer needed them rather than putting them back where they belonged. He wanted to make returning them to their designated place an automatic behavior. A method he used was to lay a yellow card under the items he would be using throughout the day. When he was done with an item, he placed it back on the card on which it had rested, therefore in its place and set to be easily found the following morning.

> *When you identify features important for automaticity, highlight and incorporate them into your practice sessions.*

Repetition

The more you engage in an activity, the more likely it can replace a senior moment.[6] For example, I spent countless hours looking for common objects such as my keys, cell phone, and wallet. At least once a month, my wallet dropped out of my pocket when I left my car. Daily, my cell phone played a hiding game with me, often resulting in me missing important calls. And my keys would often find a home between couch cushions. Without repetition, new behaviors and patterns may disappear because of the cognitive load placed on the brain.[7] We can learn much from virtuoso musicians. Vladimir Horowitz, the great pianist, still practiced scales between four and eight hours a day well into his eighties.[8]

The beauty of repetition is that it leads to automaticity, allowing the brain to retrieve a pattern with little thought. That allows the brain to focus on other things.[9] This marvelous and mysterious process occurs not only in musical performances but also in preparing foods, writing, catching a ball or repetitive activities. An example would be trying to execute a two-handed backhand during a tennis game minutes after learning it. My friend was so involved with remembering the steps and integrating them that she was not aware that every time she prepared to execute a backhand, her opponent snuck up to the net. When her tennis partners gathered, many of their comments involved a comical scene of my friend methodically preparing to hit the ball as her opponent made ready to smash it back. They incorrectly labeled her inattention a "senior moment" rather than the result of executing behaviors not yet automatic.

Contrast using a newly learned backhand with what someone can bring to the game after daily practice for a week. To effectively use a two-handed backhand, my friend needed to perform a pattern that involved at least seven sequenced behaviors:

1. Determine if the ball coming to you is for the backhand side

2. Step up into position

3. Change grip

4. Pull racket back level

5. Swing level

6. Follow through

7. Step forward

Every day she practiced the sequence for twenty minutes. By the end of the week, the pattern had been set in her long-term memory. Although it was not yet fully automatic, her brain did not need to focus as much on the sequence. This is like the Zen archer who does not think about his target after years of training. While my friend still needed to give the stroke mechanics some attention, as her swing became more automated with practice, she was able to develop more awareness of her opponent approaching the net.

Consistent Practice

How often did you think that not practicing a behavior for a short time would not have any affect, but found when you restarted, the loss of competency was more dramatic than you could have imagined? The need for consistent practice regardless of whether it is remembering names, finding objects, engaging meaningfully, or any other behavior is based on how the brain handles new information.[10] Until a behavior becomes automatic, it is fragile; its strength diminishing with time. Inconsistent practice before a behavior becomes automatic is the surest way of losing it.

Regardless of the methods you use to change a senior moment to one that will replace it, it should be practiced consistently.

TESTING FOR AUTOMATICITY

Until practice supports are removed, you will not know if a behavior has become automatic. To better understand how behaviors become automatic, identify one behavior you repeatedly do. For me, it is making coffee. I found there is no variation in the steps I perform. I scoop the coffee the same way, tap the scoop the same number of times, etc., etc. How is it possible that with minimal cognitive effort, the coffee-making process flawlessly repeats itself with little or no variation whether I am alert or groggy? The secret lies in the brain's ability to store entire patterns.[11]

When I began using a single-cup approach to making coffee, my brain began laying down the pattern. As I prepared more and more cups, the pattern became more embedded. Eventually, it became neurologically established, and with the first step (e.g., scooping beans), the brain says, "Okay, I'm ready to execute the coffee-making pattern." Not as impressive as Curry's fifty-foot shots, but just as satisfying. Once you believe your pattern has become automatic you can determine its stability by **(1) gradually removing supports and (2) testing for decay.**

Gradually Remove Supports

Sometimes we are so delighted by the change in our behaviors that we are reluctant to give up the supports that brought us to them.[12] The biggest problem is that unless you allow the behavior to occur without support, you will never know if it has become automatic. In our discussion of the client who spent hours trying to find objects, as long as he relied on the yellow cards to prevent a senior moment, he would not know if the behavior had become automatic. That would require the removal of all cards to see if the delinquent objects decided to once again hide.

Although you may be reluctant to give up supports for a behavior you now successfully exhibit, do it. Unless the behavior has a chance to go solo, you will never know if it has firmly become a part of your repertoire.

Testing for Decay

The brain's ability to retain patterns is flawed.[13] While some patterns are retained forever without practice, like learning as a child not to touch a hot stove, others, like not scanning written material may start to disappear after a few months of neglect. Pinpointing a specific number of days for an action to become automatic is impossible. But there are certainties. For example, the more you practice:

1. the quicker the behavior or pattern develops,

2. the less cognitive effort is required to execute a behavior,

3. the more robust the behavior or pattern, and

4. the longer the behavior or pattern lasts.

It makes more sense to think of the development of automatic behaviors as falling along a continuum rather than being established after a specific number of days. As the behavior becomes more automated, there is a corresponding drop in the mental effort required. The relationship between practice and the development of automatic behaviors is straightforward: The more you practice, the more likely the behavior will become automatic. The more automated a behavior, the less mental effort required to perform it. The less mental effort needed, the less likely it will lead to a senior moment.

There is no strict cutoff time for determining when a new behavior becomes stable. However, we know some relationships do exist: The more you practice a behavior, the quicker stability will be established; it takes less time for a simple behavior to become automatic than a complicated one.

Part III

The Extras

Now that you have learned how various strategies and methods can prevent senior moments, it is time to explore how variables such as self-defeating attitudes, poor sleep, and inadequate nutrition can throw a wrench into your best efforts. Finally, I'll ask you to think about what you can do if some senior moments are predictors of an uncertain cognitive future.

Chapter 12

Attitudes Needing Adjustment

If the Martians ever find out how human beings think, they'll kill themselves laughing.

—Albert Ellis

Although you may disagree with this psychologist's assessment of how bizarre human thinking is, you probably concur that we are addicted to telling ourselves crazy things and then believing they are true. Known as self-fulling prophesies, rock-solid convictions, core values, cognitive dissonance, and other phrases, they act as zealots constantly trying to direct your brain to think "the right way," which is rarely the right way.

In addition to the myths about senior moments explained in Chapter 1, here are five that I found to be most damaging to clients when they tried to create a life without senior moments: **(1) I'm always, or usually right, (2) going beyond a threshold is the way to change, (3) I just want to get rid of the senior moment, (4) I will only accept the best, and (5) all I need to change is motivation.**

I'M ALWAYS RIGHT, OR USUALLY RIGHT

I posted a scathing review when I received what I thought was a defective product from an Internet purchase. After my comments were widely disseminated, I realized the product was fine; the only thing defective was my reasoning: I did not understand how to use the item because of the speed at which I repeatedly read the directions. We all face the danger of believing our current information processing ability is as good as it was in the past. More challenging to our ego is accepting that errors often lie with us. To avoid the embarrassment I experienced you can **(1) initially assume you are wrong and (2) fact-check before you make conclusions.**

Initially Assume You Are Wrong

We have so much invested in being "right," that it may be difficult acknowledging we may have been wrong. But vehemently believing that you are right closes the door to preventing senior moments. Why change if the feedback your friends and family are giving is wrong? Studies have shown that a willingness to assume you made an error has long reaching positive effects beyond developing a more humane attitude: it can lead to greater change even if eventually you find that you were right.[1] By assuming you are wrong you become willing to explore strategies and methods of preventing a senior moment. If you adamantly believe you are right, then the door to change is closed.

Fact-Check Before You Make Conclusions

There is a psychological condition called "cognitive dissonance" that has a direct relationship on attitudes that interfere with preventing senior moments. Basically, it states that when one's beliefs conflict with actions, a tension is created and the mind will attempt to resolve the dissonance, often by accepting beliefs over facts.[2]

One vivid example is the conflict created between continuing to smoke even though there is an abundance of evidence that smoking is harmful.[3] The argument goes like this:

1. I smoke (a behavior).

2. I've read and listened to scientists asserting that smoking is unhealthy.

3. In order to resolve the conflict (dissonance) between continuing to smoke or stopping I need to choose between the scientific evidence (facts) and my need to continue smoking.

4. I decide to continue smoking because I believe the research is inconclusive (belief).

It may appear that the logic here is faulty, just as it is when election deniers explain a candidate's loss because of corruption—without evidence—rather than accepting their candidate lost because more people voted for their opponent. Siding with beliefs rather than facts can also happen with senior moments. Examine the facts before reacting when someone provides feedback to you about a senior moment.

GOING BEYOND A THRESHOLD IS THE WAY TO CHANGE

There's an old joke about a man who goes to a doctor and says, "Doctor, it hurts when I do this," moving his arm in a circle. "How can I make it better?" The doctor ponders his patient's concerns and says, "Well, don't do that." This classic joke becomes a guideline for thresholds: It is more critical to succeed by doing less than failing by attempting to exceed a threshold.[4] As we age, many of our body's systems stop functioning as they did when we were younger. When I was in my thirties, I ran a marathon in four and a half hours; not particularly fast, but for me a significant accomplishment. I still run at age seventy-seven, but people who are walking routinely pass me because I have adjusted my pace so I never exceed 75 percent of my maximum heart rate—my threshold for running without jeopardizing my health.

Many of us routinely underestimate. We offer deadlines on finishing tasks that are not even close to the amount of time it will take. We tell someone we will meet them at a specific time and then leave them waiting for us in the rain. And my favorite, believing a contractor when he tells me a whole house remodel will take only three months.

Exceeding thresholds often results in senior moments. We constantly engage in activities where thresholds are exceeded. Some are simple to spot, such as driving too long without taking a break, playing the second set of tennis when you are exhausted after the first one, and attempting to accurately write checks after spending two hours on bookkeeping. But others, such as continuing to argue beyond the point when damage to relationships is irreparable are more difficult to identify when they are occurring. You can set barriers for thresholds in the areas of **(1) physical activities and (2) cognition**.

Physical Activities

I have played handball—off and on—since in high school. Until I was in my fifties, the idea of slowing down was unimaginable. If I was interested in a slow exercise, there was always croquet. My handball playing, like my musicianship, was okay but not stellar. I was a low B player in rankings from A to C. As I aged, I still thought of myself as a B player, despite a growing midsection, a less-than-successful hip replacement, and slower reaction times. In my sixties, I continued to play with folks in their thirties as if I was their age. The result? The most enjoyable sport in my life became the cause of excruciating pain on a weekly basis. That changed when I met eighty-seven-year-old Rudy Stadlberger.

Rudy was a legend in San Francisco and throughout the handball world. He was competitive for fifty years and won numerous tournaments, including thirteen national championships. After watching me struggle playing singles with someone half my age, Rudy asked me to join him and two other octogenarians for their weekly doubles game. I had two conflicting emotions. The first was depression; believing my playing must have been so terrible that Rudy thought I was ready to play with *really* old people. The second emotion was trepidation playing with an icon, even one in his eighties.

Rudy's classic moves were still there but performed at half-speed. He appeared to analyze every shot: *Is this worth doing? What do I risk attempting the move?* I, however, was less judicious. I went for every shot, even those I knew were beyond my ability—a mistake ripe for creating a senior moment. Rudy explained that the key to his longevity was realistically accepting what he could and could not do. On the other hand, I was willing to risk injury to protect my ego. Rudy played handball into his early nineties by making wise decisions. I stopped playing in my sixties when my foolish moves resulted in physical pain and stories about the delusional "older" handball player who got "whopped" by Rudy.

For physical activities, set a threshold way below what you think you are physically capable of doing. This can either involve the speed at which you do the activity, the length of time you engage in it or only playing with people at or below your physical ability.

Cognition

We like to think that our cognitive ability is just as keen as it was twenty years ago, that our execution of a cognitive task has not been compromised by age. For some tasks, both simple and complex, that may be true; but for others, this illogical belief can lead to senior moments. For example, if your ability to follow instructions decreases when you are tired, you may want to limit your bridge games to the morning or afternoon when you are cognitively more alert. Thresholds, in this case, would involve time: If you become tired by 6:00 p.m., cut off your playing at 4:00 p.m.

I had a client who prided herself on constantly crossing thresholds, whether that involved the length of time she would exercise, going past a target point during a hike, or working on a document until she fell asleep while reading. For her, exceeding thresholds was a badge of honor, showing she still "had it" despite turning sixty-five. Exceeding thresholds was such a part of her personality that I had to suggest limits for many activities. I started by asking her how long it would take to do each activity she had scheduled for the following week. I then added 25 percent to each activity.

Once you think you have determined a threshold, assume you have overestimated your abilities and reduce it significantly. You can always bump it up later.

ACTING AS IF SENIOR MOMENTS ARE ISOLATED EVENTS

All senior moments have a history. For example, I have lived in the same house for almost forty years. For thirty of those years, I stored kitchen garbage under the sink. When we remodeled ten years ago, the contractor moved the place for the garbage can, which had been under the sink, to another cabinet a few feet away. Although 90 percent of the time I open the correct cabinet for garbage, 10 percent of the time, I still grab hold of the door under the sink. Why? Trace memory elements still exist of the garbage area before the remodel.

An understanding of the power of associations, such as my kitchen example, are used by some of the country's most effective psychologists: advertising executives responsible for developing commercials. If you examine any advertisement on television, you will realize that a product is rarely sold just on its merits. It is associated with a type of person, idea, or activity the advertiser believes will make it more desirable to a broad audience. The Mercedes Benz company advertises its cars not just as a way of transporting you from home to the supermarket, but as a symbol of celebrity status, freedom, wealth, etc. Watch advertisements for care facilities and see how they push the relief our children will experience knowing we are taken care of.

Associative strategies work because successful advertisements create connections between products or services and what advertisers believe the public yearns for.[5] To firmly wedge it into your memory, they will repeat the product name at least six or seven times within a minute or less. Think about why you found a certain advertisement appealing or why you bought a product after watching an ad. Understand that and you will understand why some inexplicable senior moments keep reoccurring.

ONLY ACCEPTING THE BEST

Several years ago, I gave a workshop on change. A participant said he was extremely distraught about a decision he was struggling for months to make—whether to vacation in Paris or London, two cities he loved. He acknowledged that no matter which one he chose, he and his family would have a wonderful time, but he wanted to determine which was "the best" and was willing to spend a lot of money and seven days to accomplish that goal by attending my workshop on change.

We often try to make meaningful decisions using ridiculous criteria, especially when distinctions are insignificant. And in the pursuit of "the best," we create senior moments. Research shows that the finer the distinctions between choices, the less meaningful they are.[6]

Do not agonize over decisions about which methods to use to replace a senior moment. Select one that is effective and acceptable, do not spend much time on determining which is "the best."

CHOOSING UNREASONABLE GOALS

You can make your goals more achievable by **(1) making them obtainable, (2) breaking them into smaller units, or (3) avoiding inappropriate goals.**

Making Goals Obtainable

Years ago, a dream fishing trip almost became a disaster. I had effortlessly waded the McCloud River in California for many years, stalking wild trout in fast water. I returned after an absence of fifteen years and expected to have the same experience that nourished my soul when I was younger.

As I looked out over the fast-moving water on a sunny July morning, I remembered effortlessly walking on rocks as I searched for the telltale movement of trophy-sized rainbow trout hovering behind boulders. Many physical changes had occurred since my last visit. Meniere's syndrome (equilibrium problem) compromised my balance, prostate cancer treatments reduced my stamina, and yes, I was twenty years older. But I disregarded these "inconsequential" changes when I decided to fish this legendary river.

I arrived early in the morning and began wading toward a riffle where I could silently cast my fly—a Goldberg Wooly Bugger. My thoughts focused on catching and releasing trophy fish as I did in the past instead of watching where I stepped. I stopped reminiscing when I was knee-high in midstream. Rocks which once posed few problems were now as slick as an oil-covered road. Even with a wading staff, I struggled to keep my feet on top of football-sized rocks covered with algae. I grew weaker, trying to remain upright, eventually falling into the fast-moving water. Wet, exhausted, and humiliated; I stumbled for thirty yards toward the shore. Without the energy or balance on top of the rocks, my feet effortlessly slid onto flat gravel beds, and I remained upright until reaching the riverbank.

Too tired to move on and too apprehensive about going back into the river, I sat on the ground feeling stupid for believing I could do something I did twenty years ago. Foolish for thinking someone suspended the aging process for me. And delusional for ignoring the changes in my physical condition. As I searched for answers for how to age gracefully, I realized the river had already provided an answer. "Adapt, Dummy," the river said. "Allow who you've become to shape how you achieve goals."

Adaptation meant I must stop clinging to the past. I went back into the river and allowed my feet to slide off the rocks onto flat gravel beds. And that was the lesson, not only for the rest of my fishing trip but also for aging. Stop struggling and adapt.

Unreasonable goals can cause senior moments. As much as you would prefer to do activities that until now never resulted in senior moments, it may no longer be possible.

Breaking Goals into Smaller Units

There is nothing wrong with having blockbuster objectives. A few well-chosen ones can act as goalposts for your life, giving it direction.[7] However, the problem with having a "big picture" objective is that it most likely will take a long time to achieve. For example, early in a person's career, a woman set her sights on becoming her company's CEO. An excellent objective, but one that might take ten years and multiple steps to achieve. What kind of reinforcement will she receive while pecking away at the ten-year career path? Wisely, she constructed monthly goals, easily achievable and each moving her ten-year goal closer.

At times a goal can be attained by changing the path toward achieving it.

Avoiding Inappropriate Goals

Stress can also result from the selection of inappropriate goals. As my sleep deprivation grew, I pretended that with "grit" I could function as I did before my nightly sleep dipped below four hours. I did not modify my exercise schedule, I committed to at least one workshop a month, agreed to family vacations squeezed between professional responsibilities, and I pretended everything was fine, despite the stress I began to experience. Even as my mental and physical health deteriorated, I vowed to myself to push forward. Eventually, feedback from my family stopped my insanity. As I changed my behaviors—reducing the number of activities and commitments—my stress level dropped. And as it lowered, behaviors that appeared to be senior moments diminished.

Choosing inappropriate goals can create stress, which can lead to senior moments. Goals should be appropriate in number and difficulty.

Believing Motivation Is Sufficient for Preventing Senior Moments

Several years ago I enrolled in an expensive cycle training program that promised I would become fit in sixty days, decrease my cycle times by 30 percent, and live longer. I think implicit in the motivational speech was that my sex life would improve, and I would grow more hair. After a pep talk by one of the trainers, I spent thirty minutes with the instructor determining my exact cycling positioning. Then he directed me to the "conditioning studio" where high-tech stationary bikes, placed in a semi-circle, faced a thirty-something-year-old instructor who could have passed as an *Esquire* model. I looked around and saw ten other cyclists who appeared to be less than half my age (sixty-five at that time) and were quickly pedaling without even sweating. I had visions of the instructor calling my wife after the session with the news that I had died on the bike and asking if she would like to purchase it as a remembrance as if it was a memorial candle.

After the class—one of the most painful experiences of my life—I asked the instructor if there was an alternative way of training. Something more sensible, possibly a routine that would not cause a heart attack.

"Motivation, Stan," he said. "That's all it takes. With it you can do anything. Without it you fail."

I nodded as if I agreed and asked for a refund. Motivation is ephemeral and rarely enough by itself to prevent senior moments. Couple motivation with knowledge and you have a powerful combination for change. Rely just on motivation, and you commit to change without knowing how to do it.

CHAPTER 13

Sleep

Sleep that soothes away all our worries. Sleep that puts each day to rest. Sleep that relieves the weary laborer and heals hurt minds. Sleep, the main course in life's feast, and the most nourishing.

—WILLIAM SHAKESPEARE[1]

HOW OFTEN DID YOU HOPE SHAKESPEARE'S VISION OF SLEEP would replace your nighttime battles? While teaching at San Francisco State University, I hoped for just a taste of the nourishment Shakespeare professed sleep could give. Unfortunately, it was as remote as my dream of playing first base for the Yankees. When I was in my mid-fifties, a twenty-five-year history of sleep deprivation became acute. There were some weeks when I never had more than three to four hours of sleep a night. After I delivered a three-hour lecture during an exceptionally difficult sleep week, my graduate assistant entered my office and wanted to talk about what just had happened.

"Did I say something inaccurate or insensitive?" I asked, knowing my sleep deprivation was affecting my teaching.

"No," she replied.

I relaxed, thinking, *no embarrassing senior moment this time.* I hoped the research literature showing that sleep depreciation affects cognition was wrong, or did not pertain to me.[2] Then she said, "but it was the same lecture you gave last week, almost word for word—even the same jokes."

Many of my students interpreted my repeated lecture as a senior moment. I retired at fifty-seven years of age when I could not find help other than prescription sleeping pills that quickly lost their effectiveness.

What is sleep, and how is it related to senior moments? Sleep is a four-part process that restores the brain.[3] In the first stage, you are transitioning from wakefulness to sleep, which should last between five and ten minutes. Then comes stage two, where your body temperature drops, your heart rate begins to slow, and your brain shows increased electroencephalogram recordings (EEG). This stage lasts approximately twenty minutes before the brain goes into a deep sleep. Finally, you enter rapid eye movement (REM) sleep when your brain becomes more active, and your body relaxes and becomes immobilized. In this stage, dreams occur, and your eyes move rapidly. Throughout your time asleep, your brain will repeatedly cycle through REM and non-REM sleep. According to the technical personnel at the Stanford Sleep Medicine Center, I never went into REM sleep during the eight hours of my visit. That finding, along with other telemetric data, led them to conclude that I had a REM sleep disorder that was probably present for decades.

Many researchers believe the primary function of sleep is to prevent and treat illnesses.[4] During sleep, spinal fluid flows through the brain and removes buildups of amyloid-beta protein, a molecule thought to increase the risks of Alzheimer's.[5] This "washing out process" only occurs during sleep. One of my most challenging sleep periods occurred just before my sixtieth birthday. Five years later, at a gathering of friends, someone recalled moments from the party. I listened to the descriptions and laughed along with everyone. What nobody knew was that I had no recollection of any of them.

Sleep is crucial for transforming short-term to long-term memory.[6] It is thought that unless the transfer is made, large amounts of information are lost. To this day, there are other significant events in my life I cannot remember because they occurred during severe bouts of sleep deprivation. An explanation given by neuropsychologists for this phenomenon is that since the information was not moved from short-term to long-term storage areas, portions of it drop out of consciousness.[7] When the transfer does not occur or is faulty, expect an increased amount of memory issues; some of which may become senior moments.[8]

Getting adequate sleep is an essential strategy for preventing senior moments. But how much sleep is necessary? We can't be precise about this, but research suggests that healthy adults over the age of sixty-five need between seven and eight hours a night.[9] Obviously, turning and tossing all night will not be beneficial even if you remain in bed for eight hours. Much of the popular litera-ture on sleep is based on common beliefs, some well-documented, others as sketchy as a carnival barker's promise of the fantastic things that will be revealed inside the tent if you give him a quar-ter. However, one excellent book that offers scientifically based practical methods for improving sleep is Arianna Huffington's *The Sleep Revolution*, a definitive work on sleep for those who seek relief from this problem.[10]

If you have sleep issues, the first step in addressing them is through a medical professional, usually a physician who special-izes in sleep disorders. Unfortunately, since sleep disorders are on the rise, there are not enough personnel to deal with the demand. In 2020 it took eight months for me to get an appointment at Stanford. Additionally, insurance may not cover the sleep study many centers require before intervening. So, if you cannot afford a visit with a specialist, cannot wait until supply catches up with demand, or for other reasons do not wish to go the professional route, here are some methods you can use to address the problem: **(1) create a sleep environment, (2) time interventions for maximum effect, (3) meditate, (4) use sleep devices, (5) take medications, (6) exercise, and (7) plan for fatigue**.

CREATING A SLEEP ENVIRONMENT

In the past, the first line of defense against sleep disorders were medications. Unfortunately, most medications are developed to treat insomnia lasting less than two weeks. These medications warn against using the drug longer since continued use may cause addiction. What many do not stress is that after two weeks, even if an addiction has not developed, the drug begins losing its effectiveness.[11] A newer, more effective and safer approach is cognitive behavior therapy (CBT), which has been used in various fields for more than thirty years.[12]

The focus of this approach is to change thinking patterns as a way of changing behaviors that contribute to poor sleep. For example, instead of using your bed for watching TV, having dinner, reading a book, etc., use it only for sleep. By using it only for this purpose, climbing into bed triggers your brain to get ready for that first stage of sleep. Another CBT principle is to go to bed at the same time every night. When it is 10:00 p.m., the brain says, "Okay, that's my signal for shutting down." Other ways you can create a healthy sleep environment is to **(1) lower the temperature, (2) keep the noise down, and (3) keep the room dark**.

Lower the Temperature

Temperature is thought to be one of the most critical factors that affect sleep.[13] Heat exposure increases wakefulness and decreases slow-wave sleep and REM sleep.[14] The Sleep Foundation recommends an ideal temperature of sixty-five degrees.[15] You can lower the temperature by keeping a window open, replacing those heat-retaining flannel sheets and pajamas with light cotton, or turning down your thermostat.

Heat has more of a negative effect on the length and quality of sleep than cold. Strive to bring your current sleep environment temperature as close to sixty-five degrees as you can.

Keep the Noise Down

Intuitively, it makes sense that the quieter the environment, the better the sleep. Environmental noise is viewed as a significant cause of sleep disturbances because it is associated with several cardiometabolic, psychiatric, and negative social outcomes.[16] When noises reduce the quality or quantity of sleep, prepare for a day conducive to senior moments. They may not be as dramatic as mine was when I repeated the lecture but consider yourself at risk for a senior moment.

Environmental noise is a significant cause of sleep disturbances. If you can reduce or eliminate them, your sleep will improve, and the likelihood of having a senior moment the following day is reduced.

Keep the Room Dark

Your brain has a built-in clock that tells it when it is time to get moving and when it is time to sleep. This is known as the circadian rhythm, and it is controlled by light and darkness. When there is less light, the brain produces more melatonin, so you get drowsy. Keeping the room dark may signal your brain that you are ready to sleep, and it will turn on the melatonin faucet.[17] If you cannot control the room's darkness, consider using blackout curtains or a sleeping mask.

Darkness is a signal for the brain to release melatonin. Change the environment so that light entering the bedroom is minimized or eliminated.

TIME INTERVENTIONS FOR MAXIMUM EFFECT

Without an adequate amount of good quality sleep, we become prone to judgment errors, short-term increased stress, bodily pain, reduced quality of life, emotional distress, mood disorders, cognitive decline, memory disorders, and performance deficits.[18] Now the good news; sometimes it only takes a few tweaks to the timing of what you are already doing to improve the quality and quantity of sleep and avoid the litany of terrible outcomes I just mentioned. These involve decisions as to when to: **(1) ingest drugs and supplements, (2) stop eating, (3) stop drinking alcohol, and (4) stop using electronic devices**.

When to Ingest Drugs and Supplements

The importance of when to take sleep prescription and non-prescription drugs is not appreciated. The directions for most prescriptions will say something like "take before sleep." Rarely do they state how many hours before sleep. Yet knowing how long it takes a medication to begin working should determine when to stop or start various activities that will affect sleep. Start too early, and the effects of the medication are lost. Start too late, and you may toss and turn for hours before falling asleep.

You will want to time the effects of a sleep medication with the time you get into bed. For example, a client with a severe REM sleep disorder went through drugs in every class of prescription medication. His physician would put him on one sleep medication for a week and evaluate its effectiveness. When the drug did not affect his sleep, the physician moved on to another drug or increased the dosage. For five years, the process continued, leaving the patient not only exhausted but also depressed. He routinely took the medication just before going to bed and became so frustrated that it was not working, he would leave the bed within thirty minutes, grab a sandwich, and turn on the TV—behaviors that interfered with the drug's effectiveness when it started to work.

What none of the professionals he saw suggested was matching the delay in the prescription's effectiveness with the time he attempted to fall asleep. After consulting with a sleep expert, he realized that the medications he was taking for sleep took at least one hour to become effective.

As important as it is to get the correct dosage for prescription drugs, non-prescription drugs, and supplements, it is equally vital to understand how long it will take before the effects begin.

When to Stop Eating

How often have you heard that having a warm glass of milk at night with a few cookies will make you sleepy? How often have you followed that advice, even adding a few more delicious items to your nighttime snack, like chocolate? And after waking in the morning after an awful night, you wondered why falling and staying asleep were so difficult. You do not have to look any further than your milk and cookies.

Digestion consumes a lot of energy. Even if you did not have the milk and cookies before bed, that delicious steak you had for a late dinner signals your brain to rev up the various systems necessary to render it into a digestible liquid. Past research indicates that all food should be avoided three to four hours before sleep.[19] Some of the newer research suggests that the type and amount of food ingested may have a more critical effect on sleep than when it is consumed.[20] You can wade through the research to fine-tune when and what to eat before bedtime. An easier approach is to use the following guidelines for food you eat later in the day:

1. Eat early.

2. Eat light-calorie foods.

3. Eat smaller amounts.

4. East food easy to digest.

In the literature, recommendations for when to stop eating and drinking range from thirty minutes to six hours. But the most common time is three hours.[21] Anything with caffeine, including chocolate, should not be eaten or drank for at least six hours before you try to sleep. The closer you eat and drink to the time you want to sleep, the more likely digestion will interfere with the brain's need to sleep, and sleep deprivation can lead to senior moments. The variation in the number of hours not to ingest food and drink will depend upon what you ate. Digesting a green salad takes less time and effort than digesting a fourteen-ounce steak. It is not always possible to find the ideal number of hours that should elapse between eating and sleeping, and even if you could, the demands of everyday living would interfere. Just guide your decisions knowing that the more time between eating and sleeping—everything else being equal—the better the quality of your sleep and the less likely a senior moment will occur the next day.

Eating requires the body to go through several metabolic operations that are controlled by the brain. These activities will interfere with sleep. The solution is to either eat lighter at night or stop eating three to four hours before you attempt to sleep.

When to Stop Drinking Alcohol

"Let's have a nightcap" is often said when someone is trying to fall asleep. They believe an alcoholic drink right before bedtime will help relax them enough to fall asleep. It does increase sleepiness, but only momentarily. What follows is a chemical reaction in the brain that makes it harder to stay asleep.

Just how bad are the effects of alcohol on sleep? In a study examining the effects of alcohol consumed throughout the day, researchers found that low amounts of alcohol (fewer than two servings per day for men or one serving per day for women) decreased sleep quality by 9.3 percent. Moderate amounts of alcohol (two servings per day for men or one-and-a-half servings per day for women) decreased sleep quality by 24 percent. High amounts of alcohol (three or more servings per day for men or two or more per day for women) decreased sleep quality by 39.2 percent.[22] Regardless of where you might be on the continuum, the recommendation is not to have any alcohol four hours before you try to sleep.[23]

Unfortunately, most events where alcohol is served are in the evening, making it difficult to abstain when a party begins at 7:00 or 8:00 p.m. Dinner for most people does not happen until at least 5:00 or 6:00 p.m., except in locales where seniors flock to early-bird specials at 4:00 p.m. You may not want to pass up a world-class chardonnay with dinner or a martini at a party. In that case, being aware of the effects of alcohol on sleep may prepare you for the next day. That awareness may be sufficient to minimize the possibility of a senior moment, if not to prevent it. It is easy to attribute senior moments to someone who may have had one too many drinks. While embarrassing behaviors may occur when one's blood alcohol rises, the cause of the senior moment may be less direct. A lack of sleep the previous night caused by alcohol may be why you cannot remember a person's name at a party, not because you drank two martinis.

While any amount of alcohol will affect sleep, the less consumed, the less effect on sleep. If possible, stop imbibing alcohol four hours before you attempt to sleep. If not, become more vigilant of your behavior the next day.

When to Stop Using Electronic Devices

You have just snuggled into bed and decided to read a new book on your tablet or watch Jimmy Kimmel hoping a boring guest will put you to sleep. After an hour or so, you finally fall asleep, but the next day you still feel exhausted after being in bed for eight hours. You followed my suggestion about not eating or drinking too close to bedtime to no avail. What happened?

Most modern electronic devices use light-emitting diodes (LEDs). Although wonderful for producing clarity and illumination on cell phones, TV monitors, computers, and tablets, LEDs play havoc with your circadian rhythm—your inner clock that tells your brain when it is time to sleep and wake.[24] Melatonin is a hormone produced in response to darkness. It signals the brain that it is time to sleep. But that is not the message the brain receives after one hour of viewing a device. The light from that device deceives the brain, making it think it is still daytime and you are not getting ready to sleep but rather preparing for "awake" activities. When should you stop viewing? There is a general agreement that you should stop at least thirty minutes before sleep. Some research shows that the effects of these light-emitting electronic devices can be neutralized by wearing inexpensive glasses that filter the light.[25]

> *Do not look at any modern electronic devices two hours before sleep without viewing them through glasses that cancel the effects of the light-emitting diodes.*

MEDITATION

Meditation is a valuable method of increasing focus. Chapter 9 contains an extensive discussion on it.

> *There are many forms of meditation. All have the same purpose, to rid the mind of thoughts. "Flushing" them out*

improves sleep quality and makes it less likely senior moments will occur the next day.

SLEEP DEVICES

Various devices are available to compensate for problems sleeping. While none correct the cause of your sleep problem, they can be used indefinitely to compensate for them. Some can be purchased over the Internet; others require a prescription from a professional. The most common ones are **(1) noise maskers, (2) weighted blankets, (3) CPAP machines, and (4) implants.**

Noise Maskers

Noise maskers generate noise that can block out environmental sounds. The masker, either in the form of a hearing aid or a pillow speaker, can reduce the effects of noise. Some maskers issue white noise, a sound that can mask an extensive range of frequencies, while others are matched to the frequencies of the noise that are most bothersome. Although all of these can be purchased without a prescription, you may wish to consult an audiologist who specializes in sleep disorders for suggestions on which maskers are most appropriate for you.

> *Noise maskers can be effective devices if they are tolerated. The problem is that you are tackling a noise problem by introducing a different type of noise.*

Weighted Blankets

A weighted blanket is helpful if poor sleep is caused by stress, anxiety, or a REM sleep disorder. The blankets come in various weights, from ten to twenty-five pounds. According to their manufacturers they use deep pressure stimulation, which boosts the hormone serotonin, reduces cortisol (the stress hormone), and increases melatonin. Manufacturers advertise that by distributing an even amount of weight and pressure across the body, the blanket calms the fight-or-flight response and prepares the parasympathetic nervous system for sleep. I have no idea if any of their claims are accurate, but I use one to prevent my nighttime thrashing caused by a REM sleep disorder from injuring my wife.

Weighted blankets are an inexpensive way of addressing a sleep disorder. Additionally, it offers protection to your partner if you thrash in your sleep, an associated feature of some sleep disorders.

CPAP Machines

Sleep apnea is a common condition in which your breathing stops and restarts many times throughout the night, preventing you from getting enough oxygen. The most common diagnostic behavior is snoring, although you can have sleep apnea without snoring. The gold standard for sleep apnea is the CPAP machine (continuous positive airway pressure). The machine uses a hose connected to a mask or nosepiece to deliver constant and steady air pressure, keeps your airway open, and helps you breathe while you sleep.

A CPAP machine is not a magic bullet, and long-term use of CPAP machines may be limited because of discomfort. Before discontinuing or rejecting a CPAP, try various masks.

Implants

An alternative to the CPAP machine is an implant called Inspire. According to the manufacturer, Inspire works inside your body while you sleep. It is a small electronic implant placed in the body during a same-day, outpatient procedure. When ready for bed, you click the remote to turn it on. While you sleep, low electrical impulses open the airway, allowing for more normal breathing resulting in better sleep. Inspire requires an assessment from a medical doctor who specializes in sleep disorders.

The long-term effects of Inspire have yet to be determined.

MEDICATIONS

Go into any drugstore and you will find shelves full of non-prescription sleep medicines. Behind the pharmacist's window are probably an equal number of prescription sleep medications. Visit any legal marijuana dispensary and you will find numerous edibles and pre-rolled cigarettes with catchy names related to sleep. Do a search on the Internet and thousands of sites pop up offering you the night-time bliss found in Shakespeare's description of sleep. It appears that there are sufficient pills available to treat the world's insomnia problems. But you may ask, if all of these prescription, non-prescription, supplemental medications, and cannabis-infused items work as the advertisers promise, why do new ones appear each year?

Prescriptions

Most sleep disorder clinics warn against using prescription drugs regularly. Yet, in 2021 more than nine million people took prescription medications for sleep. Prescription drugs fall into five categories:

1. "Z" Sedative-Hypnotics

2. Benzodiazepines

3. Dual Orexin Receptor Antagonists

4. Melatonin Receptor Agonists

5. Antidepressants

Each has different effects on the brain. In her book, *The Sleep Revolution*, Arianna Huffington wrote, "sleeping pills aren't the solution to our sleep-deprivation crisis—they're another crisis masquerading as a solution, offering a false promise that takes us further from the benefits of real, restorative sleep."[26]

While some prescription drugs will have positive effects on the quantity and quality of sleep, most are susceptible to a phenomenon known as "adaptation." Adaptation refers to how the brain deals with the effects of the drug. Just as some viruses learn to accommodate and make the body's attempts to kill them less effective, the brain does the same with drugs attempting to help it sleep. On most prescription sleep medication, there is a warning about not taking a drug for an extended period. The warning is that, after a specific number of days, you may begin developing a dependence, it will lose its effectiveness, or other side effects will occur.

There may be times when prescription sleep medication is required for more than a few weeks, such as following a traumatic emotional event or physical injury that makes it difficult to fall or stay asleep. Other situations may involve waiting for an appointment at a sleep disorders clinic where long-term solutions can be found. When I shared my concern with a physician about adaptation, she suggested I switch between sleep medications in different drug classes. Switching did help, but after two months, neither remedy was effective.

There may be occasions when the only or best possibility of sleeping is with prescription drugs. When that happens, work with your physician to prevent adaptation from occurring by alternating classes of drugs or designing a schedule (e.g., every other day) that facilitates long-term use.

NON-PRESCRIPTION DRUGS, HERBAL REMEDIES, SUPPLEMENTS, AND CANNABIS

Your drugstore is likely flooded with non-prescription drugs, many of which have not been tested or approved by the Federal Drug Administration (FDA) other than for safety. Most have a proprietary formula that includes a variety of ingredients that *may* facilitate sleep. Before using them, it is advisable to check with your physician or sleep specialist since some can interfere with prescription drugs used for other problems.

Many herbal remedies have been touted to increase the quantity and quality of sleep, ranging from lavender oil placed on one's pillow to valerian root tea. Although their effectiveness may lack solid scientific evidence, many swear by them. I am reminded of astrophysicist Carl Sagan's famous quote, "The absence of evidence is not evidence of absence."[27]

Cannabis products are currently legal in twenty-one states and Washington, D.C. While adherents of cannabis products cite anecdotes to support their claims about the effectiveness of cannabis, few carefully controlled experiments have been done, since until recently, its use was illegal and federal research money was prohibited. The active ingredients in cannabis-infused products for sleep are THC (tetrahydrocannabinol), CBD (cannabidiol), and CBN (cannabinol). There are as many combinations of these chemicals as there are products. Hopefully future research will determine the more effective combinations of these chemicals.

Since non-prescription drugs and supplements have few federal efficacy requirements other than safety, decisions about which to take may be based more on personal conviction and advertising than scientific evidence.

EXERCISE

Regular exercise improves many things, including sleep. The research found that exercise is even more important to older people.[28] What has been given less study is if the timing of exercise affects sleep. The conclusions from the Johns Hopkins School of Medicine are mixed.[29]

When to Engage in Aerobic Exercise

Regular exercise may improve sleep.[30] Why is still speculative. While many conclude that it tires out the body, so the mind craves sleep, this might be too simple of an explanation. We know that aerobic exercises get your heart pumping. They are known as "cardiovascular," or "cardio," and release chemicals called endorphins. These chemicals can keep some people awake. The suggestion is that they should exercise at least one to two hours before going to bed. This allows the endorphin levels to drop before one tries to sleep.

Exercise also raises the core body temperature, signaling the body clock that it's time to be awake. The core body temperature drops after thirty to ninety minutes, facilitating sleepiness. For other people, the effects of exercise make no difference if it happens in the early morning, midday or, in evening—exercise, no matter when it occurs, will be beneficial for sleep. The folks at Johns Hopkins had two conclusions about exercise: Exercise during any part of the day was better than no exercise, and if you want to determine when to exercise, listen to your body.[31]

Exercise can help sleep patterns if it does not encourage the production of chemicals that stimulate wakefulness. To avoid this, exercise earlier in the day.

Plan for Fatigue

Sometimes, despite our best efforts to create conditions conducive to sleep, we cannot. A work assignment may require late-night efforts, or you desperately want to watch a TV show that begins close to your desired bedtime, etc. If you know the probability is high that you will not get a good night's sleep, plan to compensate for your fatigue the next day by **(1) taking a nap and (2) scheduling for drowsiness.**

Afternoon Nap

Napping has been shown to compensate for a poor night's sleep, but its positive effects are not long-lasting.[32] That early afternoon nap may get you through the afternoon, but it may not be sufficient to carry you through the entire day.

> *Napping is fine if the goal is to get you through the next few hours after the nap ends. However, you should not depend upon it to take you through an entire day senior moment free.*

Schedule for Drowsiness

Some days you know you will be tired and more prone to senior moments. For example, as I approached the deadline for submitting the manuscript for this book, I knew I would be rekindling my relationship with exhaustion. Instead of fighting it and probably committing several senior moments because I was perpetually sleepy, I canceled unnecessary activities. I tried to limit my activities to writing, eating, daily exercise, and sleeping whenever my eyes began closing. Not a healthy schedule for the long term, but effective for two weeks.

> *When you know certain activities will lead to fatigue, and you cannot change them, reduce or restrict your other patterns to accommodate them short-term.*

CHAPTER 14

Feeding Your Brain

Life expectancy would grow by leaps and bounds if green vegetables smelled as good as bacon.

DOUG LARSON

THROUGHOUT MY STUDENT DAYS IN COLLEGE, IT WAS DIFFICULT for my immigrant mother to explain my major to her friends. None of my choices were simple like business, pre-law, or biology. Instead, it began with philosophy.

"Philosophy, what's that?" she asked during my sophomore year.

I struggled for a simple explanation she could understand. "It's about how we think, Mom." She nodded, not wanting to know more, but wondered how I would earn a living by knowing how people think. It was the same bewilderment she expressed later when I was working on my master's degree in political theory. Then came the most difficult for her to understand; a doctorate in speech-language pathology. I heard her on the phone trying to explain to her friend what I would do with my degree. After struggling to find the right words, exasperated, she finally said, "He'll be doing something with children's tongues." There was a brief silence until I heard her say, "But he won't be the type of doctor who helps people."

Although I think I help people, I am not the type of doctor who feels comfortable making recommendations regarding hydration, nutrition, and other things ingested that can have a pharmacological effect on the brain. Yet they should be included in any discussion of the causes for senior moments since the brain is reactive to what we feed it.[1] So with that qualification, I will cite some research findings that may pique your interest in acquiring more information. A book I highly recommend that makes this information accessible is Sanjay Gupta's *Stay Sharp: Build a Better Brain at Any Age*.[2] Dr. Gupta, by the way, is not only a *real* doctor but also a neurologist. While many of his recommendations are included in this chapter, others also appear that have come from primary research sources.

HYDRATION

Remember the last time you were exceedingly thirsty? You probably became concerned about the effects of dehydration on your body. But what about your brain? With as little as a 2 percent drop, you can experience decreased attention, reduced cognitive skills, and memory problems.[3] Even mild dehydration can affect how the brain functions. You can only do one thing to keep the brain happy with its water content—stay hydrated.

How to Stay Hydrated

You have probably often heard that you should drink between six and eight eight-ounce glasses of water daily. If you line the glasses on a counter, the task appears daunting, with images of you searching for bathrooms throughout the day. Although water alone, unadulterated, is the best way of meeting the goal, there are other ways of reaching it by taking in fluids such as fruit and vegetable juices, milk, herbal teas, caffeinated drinks, and soda. You can also meet the sixty-four-ounce recommendation by supplementing your fluid intake with high-water-content foods like cantaloupe, strawberries, and lettuce.[4]

Keep your brain hydrated by drinking at least six glasses of water a day. Although plain water is best, you can drink coffee, tea, carbonated beverages, etc.

NUTRITION

Food has long been acknowledged as a building block to prevent and protect against diseases. Recently, there has been evidence that some dietary factors can have an effect on specific molecular systems and mechanisms that maintain mental function.[5] But before you load your refrigerator with blueberries or some exotic fruits found in specialty stores, you should understand the current state of research in nutrition.

There are many qualifications, and what may appear as solid evidence about the effects of certain foods, are often questioned in the discussion sections of research articles. Issues are raised about the role of various types of interactions, micro-nutrients, macro-nutrients, and metabolic homeostasis. This makes it difficult for those of us who are not nutritionists to know what foods to buy and what to avoid. To make matters even more complicated, the number of chemicals, nutrients, etc., that affect the brain seems endless. So, what should you expect in this section? Think of it as a teaser on nutrition that presents some widely known documented facts and speculations. And as stated in the fine print of television commercials, *do not take anything cited below as my recommendations for what you should put in your body or avoid.* After all, I'm not a real doctor. Now that all the legal stuff is done let us look at some possibilities.

As you read through the list below, do not take them as absolutes that will protect your cognition and prevent senior moments. Instead, you may decide to eat foods containing these preferential nutrients as a supplemental strategy for preventing senior moments. I remember watching my friend fending off his father's insistence that he should eat an apple. When my friend said, "Dad, I'm not hungry," his father responded, "You don't have to be hungry to eat an apple." So, apply the father's well-intended advice when creating your marketing list: Include as many of the foods containing nutrients that *may* help your brain to remain healthy and avoid those that *may* have a deleterious effect.

Omega-3 Fatty Acids

Omega-3 fatty acids are thought to support cognitive processes and regulate genes that are important for maintaining synaptic function.[6] Conversely, diets high in saturated fat are thought to interfere with cognitive processing.[7] While researchers have determined that omega-3 fatty acids affect the brain, they have not yet determined how. Foods cited as having omega-3 fatty acids are seafood (especially cold-water varieties such as salmon, mackerel, tuna, herring, and sardines), nuts and seeds (such as flaxseed, chia seeds, and walnuts), and plant oils (such as flaxseed oil, soybean oil, and canola oil).

Curcumin

In animal studies, curcumin has shown the ability to delay the cognitive decline that is similar to what happens in human brains with Alzheimer's disease.[8] Turmeric is a good source of curcumin.

Flavonoids

Flavonoids have been shown to improve cognitive functions in the elderly.[9] Foods containing flavonoids are coca, green tea, ginkgo, citrus, wine (red more than white), and dark chocolate.

B Vitamins

Vitamins B6, B12, and folate positively affect women's memory at various ages.[10] B12 is not available from plant products. B6 and folate are found in eggs.

Vitamin C

Vitamin C is important in preventing mental decline and is associated with improving focus, memory, attention, and decision speed.[11] It is a powerful antioxidant for fighting free radicals that can damage brain cells. It may protect against depression, anxiety, schizophrenia, and Alzheimer's disease. You can also get vitamin C from citrus, bell peppers, guava, kiwi, tomatoes, and strawberries.

Vitamin D

Vitamin D helps preserve cognition in the elderly.[12] Foods containing vitamin D are fish liver, fatty fish, mushrooms, fortified products, milk, soy milk, and cereal grains.

Vitamin E

A lack of vitamin E is associated with poor memory performance in older individuals.[13] Vitamin E is abundant in vegetable oils, nuts, green leafy vegetables, and fortified cereals. How vitamin E affects cognition is not well understood, but it is likely related to its ability as an antioxidant to support synaptic plasticity.

Folate or Folic Acid

Folate or folic acid is effective at preventing cognitive decline and dementia during aging.[14] Folate is found in eggs, spinach, orange juice, and yeast. Adequate folate levels are essential for brain function, and a deficiency can lead to depression and cognitive impairment. Folic acid supplementation can help to reduce the age-related decline in cognition.

Antioxidant Foods

The brain can be damaged by various elements that have an oxidation effect on it. One highly suspected element is polyunsaturated fatty acids. During oxidation—a necessary chemical reaction of the body—free radicals are produced. To counteract the effects of free radicals, the body produces antioxidants to neutralize them. All types of berries, coffee, green tea, broccoli, seeds, dark chocolate, and nuts contain nutrients that may protect the brain.[15]

FOODS YOU MIGHT WANT TO AVOID

We are constantly told to avoid some foods in warnings issued with the fire and brimstone of an old-fashioned traveling evangelist. Some of these warnings have a scientific basis, but the rationale for others may be backed by a philosophy such as *don't eat anything with a soul*. As you learned in Chapter 5, when you do something out of fear of punishment, as soon as the punisher is removed, the behavior disappears. So, I do not intend to make you feel guilty about the food you consume. Instead, I will share some research findings on the harmful effects of certain foods and nutrients on your brain.

Saturated Fat

Saturated fat is believed to promote a cognitive decline in seniors.[16] Foods with saturated fats are butter, ghee, suet, lard, coconut oil, cottonseed oil, palm kernel oil, dairy products (cream, cheese), and meat.

Added Sugars

The brain needs energy to function. It gets it from glucose, a form of sugar. Still, if there is too much sugar in the brain, it can affect the hippocampus—the part of the brain that controls memory.[17] Food containing high amounts of sugar include sodas, baked goods, candies, and some processed foods. You do not have to deny yourself the occasional Reese's Peanut Butter Cup or soda, just do not make "sugar" a food category in your diet.

Fried Foods

What could be more satisfying than a box of fries that brings back memories of sitting with friends in your car outside McDonald's and fantasizing about who you will be with at your high school football game? What you did not realize then was that a diet high in fried foods is linked to lower scores in learning and memory because the frying process causes inflammation, which can damage the vessels that supply the brain with blood.[18]

High-Glycemic-Load Carbohydrates

Even though high-carbohydrate foods made of refined flour do not contain sugar, your body treats them as if they do.[19] This "misunderstanding" results in converting carbohydrates to glucose that may result in a sugar high, that in many ways mimic your grandchildren's behavior following their consumption of Halloween goodies. Just as you may attribute your grandchildren's off-the-wall behaviors to too many M&Ms, your senior moments may have been rigged by high glycemic foods. Foods with a high glycemic index include potatoes, white bread, and white rice. You can find many Internet sources that provide a glycemic index that groups foods into low, medium, and high. Load up with foods that have a low glycemic index and eat fewer of those with a high glycemic index.

Nitrates

Nitrates are used as a preservative to enhance the color of cured meats like bacon, salami, and sausages. Some studies have found that nitrates may be connected to depression and move the brain toward a bipolar disorder.[20] What a price to pay for a salami sandwich! Many meat products are produced without nitrates. While they extend the shelf life of products, their absence should have little effect on their taste.

When It Is More Serious Than a Senior Moment

There are known knowns. These are things we know that we know. There are known unknowns. That is to say, there are things that we know we don't know. But there are also unknown unknowns. There are things we don't know we don't know.

—DONALD RUMSFELD[1]

REGARDLESS OF WHAT YOU THINK OF DONALD RUMSFELD, AS the Secretary of Defense under Presidents Gerald Ford and George W. Bush, his observation about knowledge and ignorance encapsulates the conflict we may experience when faced with the choice of learning the meaning of certain senior moments or allowing ourselves to remain in the dark.

Many years ago, my mother seemed distracted on her annual visit. Her vibrant and feisty nature had been changing for the previous five years. Gone were the Yogi Berra type of sayings such as "No one goes there nowadays; it's too crowded." Missing were the unequivocal judgments of right and wrong. Absent was the unintentional humor from her stripped-down descriptions of current events. Instead, she was a silhouette of who she had been. I thought of these changes as I drove home after teaching a class at the university and decided to have a long-delayed heart-to-heart talk with her about my concerns.

The house was eerily silent when I entered. On each of her past visits, there always would be cooking smells and the clanking of pots. But on that day—nothing. After searching every room, calling out "Mom" and getting no response, I raced to the back deck and found an open gate leading to a forested area. I scrambled down the rickety steps, afraid of what I might find. How would I explain my negligence to the family? They had shared concerns with me, but I tried to reassure them and myself by saying, "It's nothing to worry about. That's just Mom being Mom." Not seeing any signs of her, I started dialing 911. Before I tapped the second 1, she emerged from behind a stand of trees, disheveled, carrying a bunch of leaves and twigs.

"Mom, what are you doing?"

She smiled as if having solved a complicated puzzle.

"Straightening out the forest."

I was baffled.

"The forest looked so messy from inside the house. I thought it would be nice to clean it up a little."

"But Mom, it's a forest."

She stared at me with an expression suggesting I was not intelligent enough to understand what she was trying to explain. For years, her senior moments had been a source of hilarious stories told by family members, including me. I would have another to add—probably the best one. I thought my heart-to-heart could wait.

For ten years after that incident, I thought my mother's "straightening out the forest" was her humorous take on the world. Just another senior moment to add to an extensive list of ones that had entertained my family for years. Its deeper meaning only became apparent at her memorial when friends shared her confusion in the last years of her life with me. Although we spoke on the phone every week, we only saw each other a few times a year. Our limited contact made it possible for her to conceal other events that would have led me to interpret her "straightening out the forest" as more than a senior moment.

I did not know she was getting lost while driving in her neighborhood after dark, nor only cooked with a microwave oven since she often forgot to turn off the stove-top burners. According to my mother's friends, the strangest change was her insistence that pieces of furniture in the apartment remain exactly where she placed them. I realize now that her "straightening out the forest" senior moment may have foreshadowed Alzheimer's or another form of dementia had she lived longer.[2]

I often hear the refrain, "If I'm prone to develop Alzheimer's, I don't want to know about it. Why learn I'll have a hard life before it becomes a reality?" It is normal to be optimistic when the probability of something terrible developing is low. But what happens if you ignore the possibility that certain senior moments may be predictive of Alzheimer's or other forms of dementia? You decide to roll the dice, and up comes "snake eyes?" Unfortunately, before a professional makes a dementia diagnosis, people living with Alzheimer's will walk a lonely path for years.[3]

Yes, learning why a senior moment persists—and may grow worse—might be frightening, but knowing will enable you to **(1) modify strategies and methods, (2) troubleshoot and, (3) rule out dementia.**

MODIFY STRATEGIES AND METHODS

Life never quite goes as we want it to. And as we age, disturbing thoughts that once had been on the distant horizon now expand our "worry field" daily. We always have a choice; we can ignore these thoughts because they are too frightening or confront them head-on. If you are ready to take a look, understanding the relevance of senior moments will be helpful.

Senior moments are equivalent to a car's "low oil pressure" warning gauge. The blinking light does not explain why the oil level dropped dangerously low. Instead it is the car's general signal that says, *Something is wrong with my oil pressure! I'm not sure what it is, but I might blow up if you don't attend.* Regarding senior moments, take the same cautious approach your car does for oil pressure. Your humorous event may be the basis of a self-deprecating laugh or just some normal age-related changes you are successfully addressing by applying the strategies. But what if it is not? What if, despite your best efforts, the senior moment not only persists but is getting worse?

TROUBLESHOOTING

Many senior moments result from an aging brain whose information processing ability is normal but declining.[4] Some counselors suggest accepting these events as an inevitable part of aging. While the advice is well-intentioned, it offers little solace if you can't remember your granddaughter's name, become disorientated in a familiar neighborhood, or say something ridiculous in front of someone you are trying to impress. Should you be concerned about these senior moments? Maybe, but first, gather information about the **(1) context, (2) frequency, and (3) significance of their occurrences**.

Context

Context refers to what happens before and during a senior moment. The importance of context in understanding any event—including senior moments—is found in disciplines as diverse as eastern philosophy, jurisprudence, and physics. For example, the Dalai Lama wrote that everything arises from something.[5] Ruth Bader Ginsburg relied on context to explain her dissenting vote on a decision involving Planned Parenthood.[6] Physicist Richard Feynman believed context was critical for understanding the physical world.[7]

We often ignore context when trying to understand something. Yet context is often the most crucial variable for explaining an event. For example, context can make getting lost while driving to your favorite restaurant less alarming if you slept only a few hours and had a heated conversation on your cell phone while driving. Conversely, your disorientation should raise concerns if you have had eight hours of sleep every day for the past week, only a few things are bothering you, no one is talking to you, the radio is off, and there are no visual distractions.

Frequency

Frequency refers to the number of times you repeat a senior moment. For example, is this the first time you forgot an important appointment in years or the third time this month? One of my most concerning and reoccurring senior moments is when I go from my office to another room and cannot remember why I am there. When I shared this problem with a friend, he tried comforting me by saying, "Don't worry, it also happens to me." When I responded, "It happens to me daily," he was speechless. The more a senior moment happens, the more it should be a matter of concern. The trend (e.g., rising, flat, or falling numbers) can be important for predicting the behavior's future direction.[8] For example, in the last month, has the number of times you conflated two memories increased, remained the same, or decreased?

Significance

Objective data, such as having a family history of Alzheimer's, is a reason for concern.[9] While the connection between heredity and Alzheimer's is statistically convincing, many researchers are hesitant to make a direct connection between the two. However, your concern can go beyond objective data. It can involve uneasy feelings that senior moments reflect cognitive problems other than dementia.[10] Significance also comes from believing your senior moments are harbingers of the future. For example, you may fear that forgetting a long-time friend's name may morph into being unable to recognize a grandchild's face; the momentary confusion experienced driving to a new location may grow into becoming disorientated while walking through a familiar neighborhood or forgetting an item in a favorite recipe may develop into not remembering how to make scrambled eggs.

Significance can also be purely psychological: you may not believe forgetting the name of a favorite grandchild forecasts anything ominous. However, the pain you feel from seeing your grandchild's hurt expression is enough to warrant doing something to prevent it from happening again. *A senior moment is worthy of attention if it is significant to you, whether based on objective data, intuition, or emotions.* Significance can be tied to facts such as placing your keys in the refrigerator or not remembering your zip code. Not remembering what you were shopping for in the supermarket might be considered trivial to a friend but terrifying to you if there is a history of Alzheimer's in your family.

RULING OUT DEMENTIA

If you are concerned that your senior moments point toward Alzheimer's or other forms of dementia, it is best to be tested. Testing will not necessarily identify the cause of your memory issues, but at the very least it will establish a baseline that will enable neurobehavioral practitioners to assess in the future whether you are experiencing normal brain aging or something more concerning. To paraphrase Donald Rumsfeld, even if the unknown unknowns may be devastating, preparing for them now will render them less frightening if they become knowns.

Will any strategies or methods in this book prevent Alzheimer's and other forms of dementia? No, but it can prepare you if impaired cognition becomes a part of your future. An old Buddhist saying is, you may not be able to cover a thorny road with leather, but you can wear shoes with good soles. As a communications counselor for thirty years, I found it was easier for my clients to prepare for a debilitating condition in its earliest stage rather than waiting until it was full-blown.[11] For example, when serving hospice patients with ALS (Lou Gehrig's Disease) I knew they would not be able to speak within a few months, and their inability to discuss their fears about dying would be devastating. Instead of waiting until they were voiceless to teach them how to use a computerized communication device, I taught them to use it while oral communication was still possible. These patients were more successful in using the device than those who did not start until oral communication was a memory. They also fared better in expressing their fears about paralysis and death.

Of all the senior moments we have discussed, disorientation causes the most significant anxiety and is one of the first signs of Alzheimer's.[12] Often, the anxiety disorientation causes can be reduced by understanding the context in which it occurred. For example, a client forgot his favorite restaurant was located on a familiar street—a place he had frequented many times over the past five years. When we talked, I asked him to describe when it occurred and the context. He told me that the event occurred:

1. at 10:00 p.m. following a difficult workday,

2. after he had just finished an intense conversation with his daughter,

3. he worried about medical test results he should have received but hadn't,

4. while he was listening to the radio,

5. while he was still adjusting to a new pair of glasses.

Any of these five variables would be sufficient to cause my client's senior moment. However, instead of trying to convince him to relax, I suggested he track the behavior and let me know the next time he got lost or could not find a building on a familiar street. It never happened again. But if it did, he would have had the data to explain the disorientation (e.g., new glasses) and could maybe change one or more of his behaviors (e.g., stop listening to the radio, reduce the level of anxiety by meditating, etc.), or make an appointment with a neurologist.

When to Seek Help

We often have these strange feelings that something is wrong. We don't know what it is and would prefer just to ignore them—but we can't. And as we get older, many of those feelings relate to our cognitive ability. *Was my forgetting how to get home a senior moment or should I begin exploring locked care facilities?*

Even though some clients expected the worse, they refused to get more definitive information. Their logic was, "What's the point of knowing that I will eventually get dementia? Let me enjoy whatever I can now. I'll deal with dementia when I must." Some people may look at this reasoning as healthy. After all, why not live in the present rather than give up current happiness because there is a possibility of things heading south in the future? Many people with family members who depend upon them do not have the luxury of waiting. For them, knowing now will make the future easier, regardless of the conclusions of a neurological examination.

If you are concerned that your senior moments indicate Alzheimer's or other forms of dementia, it is best to be tested. Testing will not necessarily identify the cause of your memory issues, but at the very least, it can establish a baseline that specialists can use to determine if in the future there has been any deterioration in your cognitive abilities.

We can ignore the statistics, quake in fear, or prepare. Ignoring the statistics is a greater gamble than betting a month's rent on 00 at a Las Vegas casino. Fearing dementia needlessly restricts life. And while preparation makes the most sense, little is written on how to do that. One suggestion, taken from a Tibetan saying is to bring closer those things that are the most frightening in order to get over them.[13] In the case of dementia, that translates into planning for it—even if the odds are in favor of not contracting the illness.

Not Realizing You Have a Memory Loss

Not realizing you have memory loss—anosognosia—can be based on stubbornness or a neurological problem.[14] A client would often get into arguments with his partner when the partner insisted my client was not doing something he promised. The schism widened when my client became entrenched in believing his memory was intact. Some researchers maintain a person's insistence that a memory problem does not exist may be an early sign of dementia, especially if there is abundant evidence of memory loss.[15]

If you have been told you have a memory problem and disagree, take the observation seriously. Yes, you may have a memory problem, but as you learned earlier, there are different types of memory problems; some are just age-related, but others are not. As difficult as it may be for you to accept someone's opinion that you have a memory problem when you are sure you do not, seek a professional opinion. If you are right, the professional will determine a baseline for comparison later. If you are wrong, thank your astute observer—they helped you prepare for the future.

Statistics and Willful Ignorance

A positive approach cannot change the National Institute of Health (NIH) forecast that one in ten people over age sixty-five will develop Alzheimer's—the most common form of dementia. Even more alarming, by age eighty-five, one-third of us will have the disease.[16] As grim as these figures are, a more distressing fact is the average life expectancy following an Alzheimer's diagnosis is eight to ten years.[17] It is terrifying to imagine living with any form of dementia for that amount of time. An insensitive joke told by some people is, "Don't worry about Alzheimer's. You won't be aware enough to know you have it." But the descent into dementia is rarely quick.[18]

It was said that while Ronald Reagan began showing signs of Alzheimer's during his debate with Jimmy Carter in 1984, his death was more than twenty years later.[19] People whose loved ones developed Alzheimer's tell reoccurring stories about early memory problems. While humorous when they occurred, those senior moments developed into an integral part of a person's Alzheimer's behavioral profile. It is agonizing to think about no longer recognizing your husband's face, not remembering where you live, or forgetting how to make a toasted cheese sandwich. Ignoring the possibility that some senior moments may predict Alzheimer's is as foolish as buying a house deep in a draught-ravaged forest without fire insurance.

As a speech-language pathologist, I witnessed this type of denial by some parents of disabled children. Dread for their child's future made it frightening to consider what their five-year-old cognitively impaired toddler would require as an adult.[20] Parents who were willing to think about the future prepared their children for difficulties associated with disability. The outcomes for children of parents afraid to plan for the future were very different. Similar results occur for seniors who prepare for dementia—even if the odds are small—and those who do not. The strategies and methods you have learned in this book, while not preventative for Alzheimer's or other types of dementia, will enable you to live a better life if you are unfortunate enough to contract this disease.

PREFER WAITING?

There is a concept in economics called a cost-benefit analysis. It states *going forward should be based on the costs and benefits of doing something compared to the cost and benefits of doing nothing.*[21] Let us move this concept from economics to cognition. Do the benefits of preparing for dementia even if the odds of developing it are small outweigh the benefits of doing nothing? Absolutely! Should you ignore the possible relationship between senior moments and dementia since researchers have yet to find direct connections?[22] No.

Keep in mind that this book's strategies are appropriate for memory problems ranging from quirky to "Alzheimer's-like." For example, the creative and cognitive methods in Chapter 7 are appropriate for common short-term memory problems as well as more serious ones in Alzheimer's patients. Granted, using a strategy for mild guffaws will probably be more successful for those who are aging normally than for those suffering from Alzheimer's, but cueing strategies will be more helpful than stumbling through a dementia world without cognitive helpers.

If you do decide to make an appointment with a neurologist, know that wait times can stretch to over six months, so you may want to schedule an appointment as soon as possible. You may be glad you did.

CHAPTER 16

Frequently Asked Questions

Knowledge is having the right answer. Intelligence is asking the right question.

—ANONYMOUS

WHEN I WAS TEACHING AT SAN FRANCISCO STATE UNIVERSITY, I always looked forward to a time in my lecture when I asked students if they had questions. I found that within those questions were some of the most important ideas and concerns they had about topics ranging from motivating reluctant clients to dealing with a client's loss of language. So, in that tradition, I have included in this chapter the most frequently asked questions by my clients about their senior moments, along with my answers.

I'm forgetting more now than I did last year. Is that an advancing senior moment, or is it dementia?

That's difficult to say. If it involves just short or long-term memory, I would guess that it is just a loss of processing skills related to aging. However, if the problem affects executive functioning, that might be an early indication of dementia. If you are concerned, make an appointment with a neurologist.

I tried one strategy you suggested, and it did not work. What now?

When a strategy does not work, do not move on to another one until you assess why the first one failed. It could have resulted from the method you used to implement the strategy, or it is possible that the method was not correctly applied. If you believe it was correctly applied, choose another method listed under the strategy. If other methods do not work, it may be time to move on to another strategy.

Am I limited to using only one strategy for a senior moment?

No. It is possible to use more than one strategy at a time. Feel free to combine or modify them. Nothing is written in concrete. A mantra for this book is if it works use it. If it does not, find something that does.

I don't know where I failed in preventing a senior moment. How do I begin to determine that?

It may not be necessary to determine which information processing level failed. Sometimes, just focusing on the event is sufficient for providing you with enough information to design or modify an intervention approach.

I can't tell if my senior moment falls neatly into one of your categories or two. How do I decide?

Don't waste your time trying to make fine distinctions. Some behaviors cannot be neatly described as being in one category.

I'm having a problem implementing the Slow It Down strategy. Any suggestions?

Since the Slow It Down strategy is the most effective of all strategies, it is worth making as many modifications as necessary to make it work. For example, if you cannot slow down your speech just through self-monitoring, use a metronome to keep pace or any other device that relieves you of the burden of keeping time.

I keep choosing goals I never reach. What can I do to make them achievable?

Goals can be modified in many ways (e.g., the time required to achieve, difficulty in execution, changing settings, etc.). It does not matter what method you use to achieve your goal. What is important is that you succeed with a minimal number of failures.

It seems silly to go for easily achievable goals. Why not just go for the big one?

Going for the "gold ring" often results in many failures. Having one big success rarely outweighs the emotional cost of the failures you endured to achieve it. Keep accumulating those easy goals and, psychologically, you will be in better shape than if you failed numerous times to get the big prize.

I know patterns cause senior moments, but I can't identify them. How can I make them more obvious?

When patterns are not immediately visible, take a simple inventory of what happened immediately before your senior moment. If you have identified the culprit, it will reappear in subsequent senior moments. You can also speculate and experiment. If you think you have found the pattern but are uncertain, disrupt it and see if the senior moment reappears.

How many hooks do I need to make a memory solid?

There is no specific number of hooks needed to make memories solid. However, there are two guidelines you can use: (1) the more hooks, the easier it will be to retrieve a memory, and (2) the more sense modalities used as hooks, the easier it will be to retrieve a memory.

Will I always need to be vigilant to prevent senior moments from returning?

That question is difficult to answer. Some memories created to prevent senior moments will be retrained with minimal care. But others—those that have not become fully automatic—will eventually need a bit of retouching. A good rule of thumb is to take the plastic surgeon's approach and presume everything will eventually need some work.

You list many methods to strengthen focus. Which ones are the best?

A person who needed a hearing aid asked the audiologist which one she thought was best. Her answer was "the one you'll keep in your ears, and not in your sock drawer." The same answer applies to focus and all other strategies and methods. Do not worry about what is the best or a rank ordering of strategies and methods. If you like it and it is effective, use it.

I become distressed when I fail. Is there any way of looking at a string of failures as anything other than a negative reflection on me?

When people try to implement a program and fail, their first thought is to blame themselves. Instead, blame me. There is no way any author can plan for every eventuality. Once you no longer blame yourself, look at the failure as a diagnostic tool that can direct you to a better way of achieving your goal.

I'm unsure if what I am experiencing is a senior moment that should concern me. How can I tell if it should?

Three variables will give you the information you need to decide. The first and probably most important is does it give you concern. If it does, work on it. The second is its frequency of occurrence. If this is something that infrequently happens, ignore it. If it suggests a future problem, its pattern will appear in other behaviors. And finally, examine the context in which it occurs. Often the context will give you an indication that what seemed like a senior moment really was not.

I was able to make a behavior automatic. But after a few months, the senior moment returned. Why?

Sometimes the most effective elements for automaticity are ignored or not worked on enough. When that happens, it may appear that a behavior has become automatic—and it has—but it is not strong enough to persist. Go through your program again and continue doing it until the automaticity returns.

CHAPTER 17

Final Thoughts

SEVERAL YEARS AGO, I WAS WALKING BEHIND A TWENTY-SOME-thing-year-old couple in downtown San Francisco. My hearing then—as opposed to now—was acute enough to hear their conversation. They reduced their fast pace as they approached an elderly man slowly walking in the same direction we were. Unable to go around him they exchanged mocking expressions, then imitated the man's halting movements. Eventually, the older gentleman went into a store, and they resumed their pace. The young man turned to his girlfriend and said, "When I get that old, shoot me." If he had asked me for help, I would have been delighted to give it—even early.

Unfortunately, aging is viewed by many younger people with the same discomfort experienced when a strange uncle comes uninvited to a family gathering. Despite everyone's assurance that nobody told him about the event, he is there in all his glory, wearing a plaid mothball-smelling jacket, a striped shirt, and lime green pants. He carefully combed the few strands of remaining hair across his bald head and sat in the middle of the room waiting for a simple hello but received the same amount of attention given to a tasteless bowl of bean dip.

Why are younger people so reluctant to understand the process of aging? There's an old saying that says "we fear most that which we will become." Everyone's own embarrassing uncle is looming, peeking over the approaching horizon. Those of us who have faced west and watched the sun disappear below the horizon understand that aging is neither the bogeyman nor the doddering old fool.

There is a wonderful Zen story of a farmer who became too old to work in the fields. Not able to till the soil after seventy years of providing for his family, he spent most days sitting on the porch. His son forgot everything his father did for him. *He's useless*, he said to his wife since he was now required to do most of the farm work. After much thought, the son built a wooden coffin and told his father to get in. Meekly, the father climbed inside. The son closed the lid and dragged the coffin to the edge of a high cliff. As he prepared to drop it, he heard a light tapping from inside the coffin. Opening it, he saw his father peacefully waiting to die. With a smile, he looked up at his son and said, "I know you are going to throw me over the cliff, but before you do, toss me without the coffin. "Why?" the son asked. "It's such good wood," the father answered, "you should save it for your children when they need it for you."

As we age, our self-image becomes so important that delusions are as frequent as constipation. We look back to who we were, and think of ourselves as that same person, despite a dramatically receding hairline, inability to see our shoes, or nodding even when we don't understand. Our need to stop the aging process takes the form of inappropriate relationships, nips and tucks, pretending we're enjoying activities that tax our physical abilities, and looking into a mirror and seeing only a smooth face. We relegate aging to a hidden corner in our mind and hope it will go away, as does an annoying relative. But aging is as much a part of living as birth and death. Pretending it doesn't exist or that it has little influence on our lives is a prescription for unhappiness.

We are born, develop, reflect, age, and die. I don't think anyone has found a way to extend the sequence, no matter how much we wish for a different outcome, no matter the products we buy, the new relationships we create, or the prayers we utter. Aging is not inherently good or bad; it just IS. We can try to run away from it with the help of entrepreneurs who offer magic potions, or we can get on with the business of living and the joy of accepting our identity as an older person. Remember Popeye's take on identity: "I yam what I yam, and that's what I yam." So go forth, remember who you have been and who you have become, and if necessary, put on those Depends.

NOTES

CHAPTER 1

1. Roshi Jiyu-Kennett, *Zen is Eternal Life*, 4th ed. (Shasta California: Shasta Abbey, 2000).

2. Jaye L. Atkinson, "Senior Moments: The Acceptability of an Ageist Phrase," *Journal of Aging Studies* 18, no. 2 (May 2004): 123–142, DOI: 10.1016/j. jaging.2004.01.008.

3. Justin T. Sokol, "Identity Development Throughout the Lifetime: An Examination of Eriksonian Theory," *Graduate Journal of Counseling Psychology* 1, no. 2, article 14, (2009), http://epublications.marquette.edu/gjcp/vol1/iss2/14.

4. Henri Tajfe, *Human Groups and Social Categories: Studies in Social Psychology* (Cambridge: Cambridge University Press, 1981).

5. The Ultimate Popeye Collection (1933–1945) with 138 Original, Remastered, Uncut Cartoons & Theatrical Shorts and Loaded w/ Bonus Content! (Fletcher Studios).

6. I. M. Tallberg and G. Bergendal, "Strategies of Lexical Substitution and Retrieval in Multiple Sclerosis," *Aphasiology*, 23, no. 9 (2009): 1184–1195, DOI: 10.1080/02687030802436884.

7. Joseph R. Ferrari et al., "Frequent Behavioral Delay Tendencies by Adults," *Journal of Cross-Cultural Psychology*, 38 (2007): 458–464, DOI: 10.1177/0022022107302314.

8. Aleea L. Devitt and Daniel L. Schacter, "False Memories with Age: Neural and Cognitive Underpinnings," *Neuropsychologia* 91 (October 2016): 346–359, DOI: 10.1016/j.neuropsychologia.2016.08.030, PMCID: PMC5075259, NIHMSID: NIHMS815717, PMID: 27592332.

9. Joyce W. Lacy and Craig E. L. Stark, "The Neuroscience of Memory: Implications for the Courtroom," *Nature Reviews Neuroscience* 14, no. 9 (2013): 649–658, DOI: 10.1038/nrn3563, PMCID: PMC4183265, PMID: 23942467.

10. Brandon Berry, "Minimizing Confusion and Disorientation: Cognitive Support Work in Informal Dementia Caregiving," *Journal of Aging Studies* 30 (August 2014): 121–130. Published online June 11, 2014. DOI: 10.1016/j.

jaging.2014.05.001, PMCID: PMC4443911, NIHMSID: NIHMS594723, PMID: 24984915.

11. Vaisakh Puthusseryppady, Luke Emrich-Mills, Ellen Lowry, Martyn Patel, and Michael Hornberger, "Spatial Disorientation in Alzheimer's Disease: The Missing Path from Virtual Reality to Real World," *Frontiers in Aging Neuroscience* 12 (2020), DOI: 10.3389/fnagi.

CHAPTER 2

1. His Holiness the 14th Dalai Lama of Tibet, "In Praise of Dependent Arising—First Day," October 9, 2021, webcast, https://www.dalailama.com/news/2021/in-praise-of-dependent-arising-first-day.

2. M. Regopoulos, "The Principle of Causation as a Basis of Scientific Method," *Management Science* 12, no. 8, (April 1966), B-287–C-177, https://doi.org/10.1287/mnsc.12.8.C135.

3. Sarah Pruitt, "Why Does the Leaning Tower of Pisa Lean?" https://www.history.com/news/why-does-the-leaning-tower-of-pisa-lean.

4. Ralph Adolphs, "The Social Brain: Neural Basis of Social Knowledge." *Annual Review Psychology* 60 (January 10, 2009): 693–716, DOI: 10.1146/annurev.psych.60.110707.163514, PMID: 18771388, PMCID: PMC2588649.

5. Carol A. Seger and Earl K. Miller, "Category Learning in the Brain," *Annual Review of Neuroscience* 33 (July 21, 2010): 203–19, DOI: 10.1146/annurev.neuro.051508.135546, PMID: 20572771, PMCID: PMC3709834.

6. Eric Jonas and Konrad Paul Kording, "Could a Neuroscientist Understand a Microprocessor?" *PLOS Computational Biology* 13, no. 1, DOI: 10.1371/journal.pcbi.1005268.

7. Kåre Rumar, "The Role of Perceptual and Cognitive Filters in Observed Behavior," *Human Behavior and Traffic Safety*, eds. Leonard Evans and Richard C. Schwing (Boston: Springer, 1985), https://doi.org/10.1007/978-1-4613-2173-6_8.

8. Holly A. Ruff & Mary C. Capozzoli, "The Development of Attention and Distractibility in the First 4 Years of Life," *Developmental Psychology* 39 (September 2003): 877–90.

9. Howard Eichenbaum, *The Cognitive Neuroscience of Memory* (New York: Oxford University Press, 2002).

10. Paul W. Frankland, Sheena A. Josselyn, and Stefan Köhler, "The Neurobiological Foundation of Memory Retrieval," *Nature Neuroscience* 22, no. 10 (October 2019): 1576–1585, PMCID: PMC6903648, NIHMSID: NIHMS1061667, PMID: 31551594.

11. Aleea L. Devitt and Daniel L. Schacter, "False Memories with Age: Neural and Cognitive Underpinnings," *Neuropsychologia* 91 (October 2016): 346–359, DOI: 10.1016/j.neuropsychologia.2016.08.030, PMCID: PMC5075259, NIHMSID: NIHMS815717, PMID: 27592332.

12. Sydney MacLeod, Michael G. Reynolds, and Hugo Lehmann, "The Mitigating Effect of Repeated Memory Reactivations on Forgetting," *NPJ Science of Learning* 3, article 9 (April 2018), https://doi.org/10.1038/s41539-018-0025-x.

13. Stan Goldberg, *Ready to Learn* (New York: Oxford University Press, 2005).

14. Greg J. Stephens, Lauren J. Silbert, and Uri Hasson, "Speaker-Listener Neural Coupling Underlies Successful Communication," *Proceedings of the National Academy of Sciences of the United States of America* 107, no. 32 (August 10, 2010): 14425–30.

15. Donna J. Bridge and Ken A. Paller, "Neural Correlates of Reactivation and Retrieval-Induced Distortion," *Journal of Neuroscience* 32. no. 35 (2012), 12144–12151, DOI: 10.1523/jneurosci.1378-12.2012.

16. Nicole M. Dudukovic, Elizabeth J. Marsh, and Barbara Tversky, "Telling a Story or Telling it Straight: The Effects of Entertaining Versus Accurate Retellings on Memory," *Applied Cognitive Psychology* 18, no 2 (2004): 125–143.

17. Fergus I. M. Craik, "Effects of Distraction on Memory and Cognition: A Commentary," *Frontiers in Psychology* 5 (2014): 841, https://doi.org/10.3389/fpsyg.2014.00841.

18. Michelle E. Watts, Roger Pocock, and Charles Claudianos, "Brain Energy and Oxygen Metabolism: Emerging Role in Normal Function and Disease," *Frontiers in Molecular Neuroscience* 22 (June 2018), https://doi.org/10.3389/fnmol.2018.00216.

CHAPTER 3

1. Michio Kaku, *The Future of the Mind: The Scientific Quest to Understand, Enhance, and Empower the Mind* (New York: Doubleday, 2014).

2. Neil DeGrasse Tyson, "How Does the Brain Work?" *NOVA scienceNOW,* www.pbs.org, September 14, 2011.

3. Martin L. Lonky, "Human Consciousness: A Systems Approach to the Mind/Brain Interaction," *Journal of Mind & Behavior* 24, no. 1 (Winter 2003): 91–118.

4. Verica Vasic, Kathrin Barth, and Mirko H. H. Schmidt, "Neurodegeneration and Neuro-Regeneration–Alzheimer's Disease and Stem Cell Therapy," *International Journal of Molecular Sciences* 20, no. 17 (August 31, 2019): 4272, https://doi.org/10.3390/ijms20174272, PMCID: PMC6747457, PMID: 31480448.

5. Shaista Jabeen and Vatsala Thirumalai, "The Interplay Between Electrical and Chemical Synaptogenesis," *Journal of Neurophysiology* 120, no. 4 (2018): 1914–1922, DOI: 10.1152/jn.00398.2018, PMCID: PMC6230774, PMID: 30067121.

6. Larry R. Squire et al., "Memory Consolidation," *Cold Spring Harbor Perspectives in Biology* 7, no. 8 (August 3, 2015), DOI: 10.1101/cshperspect.a021766, PMCID: PMC4526749, PMID: 26238360.

7. Anna Christina Nobre and Freek van Ede, "Under the Mind's Hood: What We Have Learned by Watching the Brain at Work," *Journal of Neuroscience* 40, no. 1 (January 2020), 89–100, https://doi.org/10.1523/jneurosci.0742-19.2019.

8. B. F. Skinner, *Science and Human Behavior* (New York: Free Press, 1965).

9. Evan Heit, "Brain Imaging, Forward Inference, and Theories of Reasoning," *Frontiers in Human Neuroscience* 8 (January 09, 2015), https://doi.org/10.3389/fnhum.2014.01056.

10. Yee-Haur Mah et al., "Human Brain Lesion-Deficit Inference Remapped," *Brain* 137, no. 9 (September 2014): 2522–2531, https://doi.org/10.1093/brain/awu164.

11. Srimant P. Tripathy and Haluk Ö⊠men, "Sensory Memory Is Allocated Exclusively to the Current Event-Segment," *Frontiers in Psychology* 9 (September 7, 2018), https://doi.org/10.3389/fpsyg.2018.01435.

12. Ibid.

13. Nelson Cowan, "What Are the Differences Between Long-Term, Short-Term, and Working Memory?" *Progress in Brain Research* 169 (2008): 323–338, DOI: 10.1016/S0079-6123(07)00020-9, PMCID: PMC2657600, NIHMSID: NIHMS84208, PMID: 18394484.

14. Marco Cascella and Yasir Al Khalili, *Short Term Memory Impairment* (St. Petersburg, FL: StatPearls Publishing, 2022).

15. Björn Rasch and Jan Born, "About Sleep's Role in Memory," *Physiological Reviews* 93, no. 2 (April 2013): 681–766, DOI: 10.1152/physrev.00032.2012, PMCID: PMC3768102, PMID: 23589831.

16. Larry R. Squire, "Memory and Brain Systems: 1969–2009," *Journal of Neuroscience* 29, no. 41 (October 14, 2009): 12711–12716, https://doi.org/10.1523/JNEUROSCI.3575-09.2009.

17. John Jonides et al., "The Mind and Brain of Short-Term Memory," *Annual Review of Psychology* 59 (2008):193–224, DOI: 10.1146/annurev.psych.59.103006.093615.

18. Nelson Cowan, "What Are the Differences Between Long-Term, Short-Term, and Working Memory?" 323–338.

19. Jarrad A. G. Lum and Gina Conti-Ramsden, "Long-Term Memory: A Review and Meta-Analysis of Studies of Declarative and Procedural Memory in Specific Language Impairment," *Topics in Language Disorders* 33, no. 4 (December 1, 2013): 282–297, https://doi.org/10.1097/01.tld.0000437939.01237.6a, PMCID: PMC3986888, EMSID: EMS57240, PMID: 24748707.

20. Sanjay G. Manohar, Yoni Pertzov, and Masud Husain, "Short-Term Memory for Spatial, Sequential and Duration Information," *Current Opinion Behavioral Sciences* 17 (October 2017): 20–26, DOI: 10.1016/j.cobeha.2017.05.023, PMCID: PMC5678495, PMID: 29167809.

21. Alan Baddeley, "Working Memory: Theories, Models, and Controversies," *Annual Review of Psychology* 63 (2012):1–29. https://doi.org/10.1146/annurev-psych-120710-100422.

22. Fidelia Bature et al., "Signs and Symptoms Preceding the Diagnosis of Alzheimer's Disease: A Systematic Scoping Review of Literature from 1937 to 2016," *BMJ Open* 7, no. 8 (August 28, 2017), https://doi.org/10.1136/bmjopen -2016-015746.

STRATEGIES

1. Jack Welch, *Winning* (New York: Harper Business, 2005).

CHAPTER 4

1. Benjamin Franklin, *Poor Richard's Almanac* (Mount Vernon, New York: Peter Pauper Press, 1980).

2. Peter N. C. Mohr and Irene E. Nagel, "Variability in Brain Activity as an Individual Difference Measure in Neuroscience?" *Journal of Neuroscience* 30, no. 23 (June 9, 2010): 7755–7757; https://doi.org/10.1523/JNEUROSCI.1560-10 .2010.

3. B. J. Diamond et al., "Information Processing in Older Versus Younger Adults: Accuracy Versus Speed," *International Journal of Rehabilitation and Health* 5, (2000): 55–64. https://doi.org/10.1023/A:1012911203468.

4. Natasha Warner et al., "Native Listeners' Use of Information in Parsing Ambiguous Casual Speech," *Brain Sciences* 12, no. 7 (July 15, 2022): 930, https: //doi.org/10.3390/brainsci12070930.

5. A. J. Hudspeth and Masakazu Konishi, "Auditory Neuroscience: Development, Transduction, and Integration," *PNAS* 97, no. 22 (October 24, 2000): 11690–11691, https://doi.org/10.1073/pnas.97.22.11690.

6. Bong Jik Kim and Seung-Ha Oh, "Age-Related Changes in Cognition and Speech Perception," *Journal of Audiology & Otology.* 17, no. 2 (September 2013): 54–58, https://doi.org/10.7874/kja.2013.17.2.54, PMCID: PMC3936542, PMID: 24653907.

7. Karen S. Helfer, Gabrielle R. Merchant, and Peter A. Wasiuk, "Age-Related Changes in Objective and Subjective Speech Perception in Complex Listening Environments," *Journal of Speech, Language, and Hearing Research* 60, no. 10 (October 2017): 3009–3018, https://doi.org/10.1044/2017_JSLHR-H-17 -0030, PMCID: PMC5945070, PMID: 29049601.

8. Stanley A. Goldberg, *Clinical Intervention: A Philosophy and Methodology for Clinical Practice* (New York: Macmillan, 1993).

9. David B. Pisoni, "Speech Perception: Some New Directions in Research and Theory," *Journal of the Acoustical Society of America* 78, no. 1, pt 2 (July 1985): 381–388, https://doi.org/10.1121/1.392451, PMCID: PMC3517998, NIHM-SID: NIHMS418763, PMID: 4031245.

10. Jeeun Yoo et al., "Comparison of Speech Rate and Long-Term Average Speech Spectrum between Korean Clear Speech and Conversational Speech,"

Journal of Audiology & Otology 23, no. 4 (October 2019): 187–192. DOI: 10.7874/jao.2019.00115, PMCID: PMC6773961, PMID: 31319638.

11. Isabel Pavão Martins et al., "Speech Rate and Fluency in Children and Adolescents," *Child Neuropsychology* 13, no. 4 (June 12, 2007): 319–332, https://doi.org/10.1080/09297040600837370.

12. Jay Leonard, " Why Do Customers Hate Your Offshore Call Center So Much?" *Business 2 Community* (January 2023), https://www.business2community.com/customer-experience/customers-hate-offshore-call-center-much-0855971.

13. Stewart Cotterill, "Preparing for Performance: Strategies Adopted Across Performance Domains," *Sport Psychologist* 29, no. 2 (2015): 158–170, https://doi.org/10.1123/tsp.2014-0035.

14. Wammes, Jeffrey D., Brady R. T. Roberts, and Myra A. Fernandes, "Task Preparation as a Mnemonic: The Benefits of Drawing (and Not Drawing)." *Psychonomic Bulletin & Review* 25, no. 6 (2018): 2365–2372, DOI: 10.3758/s13423-018-1477-y.

15. Robert Lohmann, "Effects of Simulation-Based Learning and One Way to Analyze Them," *Journal of Political Science Education* 16, no. 4 (2020): 479–495, https://doi.org/10.1080/15512169.2019.1599291.

16. Susannah V. Levi, Stephen J. Winters, David B. Pisoni, "Effects of Cross-Language Voice Training on Speech Perception: Whose Familiar Voices Are More Intelligible?" *Journal of the Acoustical Society of America* 13, no. 6 (December 2011): 4053–4062, DOI: 10.1121/1.3651816, PMCID: PMC3253604, PMID: 22225059.

17. Fatimah Lateef, "Simulation-Based Learning: Just Like the Real Thing," *Journal of Emergencies, Trauma, and Shock* 3, no. 4 (2010): 348–352, DOI: 10.4103/0974-2700.70743, PMCID: PMC2966567, PMID: 21063557.

18. Ibid.

19. Kristian Kersting, "Machine Learning and Artificial Intelligence: Two Fellow Travelers on the Quest for Intelligent Behavior in Machines," *Frontiers in Big Data* 1 (November 19, 2018), https://doi.org/10.3389/fdata.2018.00006.

20. Mark A. Pitt, "How Are Pronunciation Variants of Spoken Words Recognized? A Test of Generalization to Newly Learned Words," *Journal of Memory and Language* 61, no. 1 (July 2009): 19–36, DOI: 10.1016/j.jml.2009.02.005, PMID: 20161243, PMCID: PMC2706522.

21. Hans Rutger Bosker, David Peeters, and Judith Holler, "How Visual Cues to Speech Rate Influence Speech Perception," *Quarterly Journal of Experimental Psychology* 73, no. 10 (2020): 1523–1536, https://doi.org/10.1177/1747021820914564.

22. Rossana De Beni, Erika Borella, and Barbara Carretti, "Reading Comprehension in Aging: The Role of Working Memory and Metacomprehension," *Aging, Neuropsychology, and Cognition* 14, no. 2 (2007): 189–212, DOI: 10.1080/13825580500229213.

23. Justine Marie Fancher, "How is Comprehension Affected When Reading Aloud Versus Reading Silently?" Education and Human Development Master's Theses (2008): 276.

24. Jinghui Hou, Yijie Wu, and Erin Harrell, "Reading on Paper and Screen Among Senior Adults: Cognitive Map and Technophobia," *Frontiers in Psychology* 8 (December 19, 2017): 2225, DOI: 10.3389/fpsyg.2017.02225, PMCID: PMC5742182, PMID: 29312073.

25. Helga Rut Gudmundsdottir, "Advances in Music-Reading Research," *Music Education Research* 12, no. 4 (December 2010): 331–338.

26. Benjamin Grindlay, "Missing the Point: The Effect of Punctuation on Reading Performance," a dissertation submitted in the Department of Psychology, The University of Adelaide (July 2002).

27. Thomas Newkirk, "The Case for Slow Reading," *Educational Leadership* 67, no 6 (March 2010): 6–11.

28. Ibid.

29. Stanley A. Goldberg, *Loving, Supporting, and Caring for the Cancer Patient* (Lanham, MD: Rowman & Littlefield, 2016).

30. Maria Klatte, Kirstin Bergström, and Thomas Lachmann, "Does Noise Affect Learning? A Short Review on Noise Effects on Cognitive Performance in Children," *Frontiers in Psychology* 4 (August 2013): 578, DOI: 10.3389/fpsyg.2013.00578, PMCID: PMC3757288, PMID: 24009598.

31. Elahe Tavakoli and Shiela Kheirzadeh, "The Effect of Font Size on Reading Comprehension Skills: Scanning for Key Words and Reading for General Idea," *Theory and Practice in Language Studies* 1, no. 7 (July 2011): 915–919, DOI: 10.4304/tpls.1.7.915-919.

32. Daniel L. Murman, "The Impact of Age on Cognition," *Seminars in Hearing* 36, no. 3 (August 2015): 111–121, DOI: 10.1055/s-0035-1555115, PMCID: PMC4906299, PMID: 27516712.

CHAPTER 5

1. Denise Fournier, PhD, "The Only Way to Eat an Elephant," *Psychology Today* (April 18, 2018), https://www.psychologytoday.com/us/blog/mindfully -present-fully-alive/201804/the-only-way-eat-elephant#:~:text=Desmond %20Tutu%20once%20wisely%20said,a%20little%20at%20a%20time.

2. Ralf C. Buckley, "Aging Adventure Athletes Assess Achievements and Alter Aspirations to Maintain Self-Esteem," *Frontiers in Psychology* 9 (February 28, 2018): 225, DOI: 10.3389/fpsyg.2018.00225.

3. Peter J. Nassiff and E. R. Boyko, "Teaching the Method of Successive Approximations," *Journal of Chemical Education* 55, no. 6 (June 1, 1978): 376, https://doi.org/10.1021/ed055p376.

4. Stanley A. Goldberg, *Ready to Learn: How to Help Your Preschooler Succeed.* (New York: Oxford University Press, 2005).

5. Stanley A. Goldberg, *Clinical Intervention: A Philosophy and Methodology for Clinical Practice* (New York: Macmillan, 1993).

6. Mark E. Bouton, "Why Behavior Change is Difficult to Sustain," *Preventive Medicine* 68 (November 2014): 29–36, https://doi.org/10.1016/j.ypmed.2014.06 .010, PMCID: PMC4287360, NIHMSID: NIHMS605603, PMID: 24937649.

7. Robert D. Sege, MD, and Benjamin S. Siegel, MD, "Effective Discipline to Raise Healthy Children," *Pediatrics* 142, no. 6 (December 2018), https://doi.org /10.1542/peds.2018-3112.

Chapter 6

1. Isaiah Berlin, *The Proper Study of Mankind: An Anthology of Essays* (New York, NY: Farrar, Straus, and Giroux, 2000).

2. Mark P. Mattson, "Superior Pattern Processing Is the Essence of the Evolved Human Brain," *Frontiers in Neuroscience* 8 (August 22, 2014): 265, DOI: 10.3389/fnins.2014.00265, PMID: 25202234, PMCID: PMC4141622.

3. Jerry L. Deffenbacher and Richard M. Suinn, "Systematic Desensitization and the Reduction of Anxiety," *The Counseling Psychologist* 16, no. 1 (June 30, 2016) https://doi.org/10.1177/0011000088161002.

4. Rick Penny, "Three Components of a Quick Release: How Stephen Curry & Melissa Dixon Use Them to Their Advantage," *Breakthrough Basketball* 13 (Oct 2022).

5. "Stephen Curry Has Hit 42.8 Percent of His Threes in His Career," *Statmuse* 15 (October 2022), https://www.statmuse.com/nba/ask/steph-curry-career -3pt-percentage.

6. "A Day in the Life: Stephen Curry," *Owaves* (June 12, 2018), https://owaves .com/day-plans/day-life-stephen-curry.

7. Lexia Zhan et al., "Effects of Repetition Learning on Associative Recognition Over Time: Role of the Hippocampus and Prefrontal Cortex," *Frontiers in Human Neuroscience* 12 (July 11, 2018), DOI: 10.3389/fnhum.2018.00277, PMID: 30050418, PMCID: PMC6050388.

8. Fuu-Jiun Hwang et al., "Motor Learning Selectively Strengthens Cortical and Striatal Synapses of Motor Engram Neurons," *Neuron Report* 110, no. 17 (July 08, 2022), DOI: https://doi.org/10.1016/j.neuron.2022.06.006.

9. Paul Seli, et al, "Intentionality and Meta-Awareness of Mind Wandering: Are They One and the Same, or Distinct Dimensions?" *Psychonomic Bulletin & Review* 24, no. 6 (December 2017): 1808–1818, DOI: 10.3758/s13423-017- 1249-0, PMID: 28244016, PMCID: PMC5572547.

10. Enamul Hoque, MD, "Memorization: A Proven Method of Learning," *The Journal of Applied Research* 22, no. 3 (2018): 142–150.

11. Kelsey, Lilly, "Chaining Techniques: A Systematic Literature Review and Best Practice Recommendations," *Culminating Projects in Community Psychology, Counseling and Family Therapy* 74 (2020), https://repository.stcloudstate.edu/ cpcf_etds/74.

CHAPTER 7

1. Ferris Jabr, "Why Your Brain Needs More Downtime," *Scientific American* (October 15, 2013).

2. Nicholas A. Bishop, Tao Lu, Bruce A. Yankner, "Neural Mechanisms of Ageing and Cognitive Decline," *Nature* 464, no. 7288 (March 2010): 529–35, DOI: 10.1038/nature08983, PMID: 20336135, PMCID: PMC2927852.

3. Verica Vasic, Kathrin Barth, Mirko H. H. Schmidt, "Neurodegeneration and Neuro-Regeneration—Alzheimer's Disease and Stem Cell Therapy," *International Journal of Molecular Sciences* 20, no. 17 (August 31, 2019): 4272, DOI: 10.3390/ijms20174272, PMID: 31480448, PMCID: PMC6747457.

4. Bryan Goodwin and Kirsten B. Miller, "Creativity Requires a Mix of Skills," *Research Says* 70, no. 5 (February 1, 2013): 80–82.

5. Eric Gorges, *A Craftsman's Legacy with Eric Gorges* (PBS), www.craftmanslegacy.com.

6. Michael W. Richardson, "How Much Energy Does the Brain Use?" Brain-Facts.org, (February 1, 2019); https://www.brainfacts.org/brain-anatomy-and-function/anatomy/2019/how-much-energy-does-the-brain-use-020119.

7. Yoed N. Kenett et al., "Driving the Brain Towards Creativity and Intelligence: A Network Control Theory Analysis," *Neuropsychologia* 118, part A (2018): 79–90. DOI: 10.1016/j.neuropsychologia.2018.01.001, PMID: 29307585, PMCID: PMC6034981.

8. Michelle E. Watts, Roger Pocock, and Charles Claudianos, "Brain Energy and Oxygen Metabolism: Emerging Role in Normal Function and Disease," *Frontiers in Molecular Neuroscience* 11 (June 22, 2018), https://doi.org/10.3389/fnmol.2018.00216.

9. Hyun-Jun Kim et al., "Effects of Oxygen Concentration and Flow Rate on Cognitive Ability and Physiological Responses in the Elderly," *Neural Regeneration Research* 8, no. 3 (January 25, 2013): 264–269, DOI: 10.3969/j.issn.1673-5374.2013.03.009, PMID: 25206597, PMCID: PMC4107523.

10. Patrick Fissler et al., "Jigsaw Puzzling Taps Multiple Cognitive Abilities and Is a Potential Protective Factor for Cognitive Aging," *Frontiers in Aging Neuroscience* 10 (October 1, 2018): 299, DOI: 10.3389/fnagi.2018.00299, PMID: 30327598, PMCID: PMC6174231.

11. Carolin Shah et al., "Neural Correlates of Creative Writing: An fMRI Study," *Human Brain Mapping* 34, no. 5 (May 2013): 1088–101, DOI: 10.1002/hbm.21493, PMID: 22162145, PMCID: PMC6869990.

12. Niklas Johannes, Matti Vuorre, and Andrew K. Przybylski, "Video Game Play is Positively Correlated with Well-Being," *Royal Society of Open Science* 17, no. 2 (February 2021), https://doi.org/10.1098/rsos.202049.

13. Denilson Brilliant T., Rui Nouchi, Ryuta Kawashima, "Does Video Gaming Have Impacts on the Brain: Evidence from a Systematic Review," *Brain Sciences* 9, no. 10 (September 2019): 251, DOI: 10.3390/brainsci9100251, PMID: 31557907, PMCID: PMC6826942.

14. Inge L. Wilms, Anders Petersen, and Signe Vangkilde, "Intensive Video Gaming Improves Encoding Speed to Visual Short-Term Memory in Young Male Adults," *Acta Psychologica* 142, no. 1 (January 2013): 108–118, DOI: 10.1016/j.actpsy.2012.11.003.

15. Laura Steenbergen et al., "Action Video Gaming and Cognitive Control: Playing First Person Shooter Games Is Associated with Improved Action Cascading but Not Inhibition," *PLoS ONE* 10, no. 12 (2015), https://doi.org/10.1371/journal.pone.0144364.

16. M. Moisala et al., "Gaming is Related to Enhanced Working Memory Performance and Task-Related Cortical Activity," *Brain Research* 1655 (January 15, 2017): 204–215, DOI: 10.1016/j.brainres.2016.10.027.

17. S. Kühn et al., "The Neural Basis of Video Gaming," *Translational Psychiatry* 1, no. 53 (November 15, 2011), https://doi.org/10.1038/tp.2011.53.

18. Giovanni Sala, John P. Foley, and Fernand Gobet, "The Effects of Chess Instruction on Pupils' Cognitive and Academic Skills: State of the Art and Theoretical Challenges," *Frontiers in Psychology* 8 (February 23, 2017), https://doi.org/10.3389/fpsyg.2017.00238, PMID: 28280476; PMCID: PMC5322219.

19. Louise F. Pendrya and Jessica Salvatore, "Individual and Social Benefits of Online Discussion Forums," *Computers in Human Behavior* 50 (September 2015): 211–220, https://doi.org/10.1016/j.chb.2015.03.067.

20. Fatimah Lateef, "Simulation-Based Learning: Just Like the Real Thing," *Journal of Emergencies, Trauma, and Shock* 3, no. 4 (October 2010): 348–52, DOI: 10.4103/0974-2700.70743, PMID: 21063557, PMCID: PMC2966567.

21. Robert C. Rubel, "The Epistemology of War Gaming," *Naval War College Review* 59, no. 2, article 8 (2006), https://digital-commons.usnwc.edu/nwc-review/vol59/iss2/8.

CHAPTER 8

1. George Carlin, *Brain Droppings* (New York: Hyperion, 1998).

2. Roland Pusch et al, "Working Memory Performance is Tied to Stimulus Complexity," https://doi.org/10.1101/2021.09.10.459776.

3. Doug Jones, *Bending Toward Justice: The Birmingham Church Bombing that Changed the Course of Civil Rights* (All Points Books, 2019).

4. Mariam Hovhannisyan et al., "The Visual and Semantic Features That Predict Object Memory: Concept Property Norms For 1,000 Object Images," *Memory & Cognition* 49, no. 4 (May 2021): 712–731, DOI: 10.3758/s13421-020-01130-5, PMID: 33469881, PMCID: PMC8081674.

5. Andrew P. Yonelinas et al., "Separating the Brain Regions Involved in Recollection and Familiarity in Recognition Memory," *Journal of Neuroscience* 25, no. 11 (March 2005): 3002–3008; https://doi.org/10.1523/JNEUROSCI.5295-04.2005.

6. Regina G. Richards, "Making It Stick: Memorable Strategies to Enhance Learning," LD Online (2008), http://www.ldonline.org/article/5602.

7. Phillip M. Tell, "Influence of Vocalization on Short-Term Memory," *Journal of Verbal Learning and Verbal Behavior* 10, no. 2 (1971): 149–156.

8. Alan D. Castel, "Aging and Memory for Numerical Information: The Role of Specificity and Expertise in Associative Memory," *The Journals of Gerontology: Series B*, 62, no. 3 (May 2007): P194–P196, https://doi.org/10.1093/geronb/62.3.P194.

CHAPTER 9

1. Paulo Coelho, *The Devil and Miss Prym* (New York: Harper One, 2021).

2. Chet C. Sherwood, Francys Subiaul, Tadeusz W. Zawidzki, "A Natural History of the Human Mind: Tracing Evolutionary Changes in Brain and Cognition," *Journal of Anatomy* 212, no. 4 (April 2008): 426–54, DOI: 10.1111/j.1469-7580.2008.00868.x, PMID: 18380864, PMCID: PMC2409100.

3. Sofie Compernolle et al., "Effectiveness of Interventions Using Self-Monitoring to Reduce Sedentary Behavior in Adults: A Systematic Review and Meta-Analysis," *International Journal of Behavioral Nutrition and Physical Activity* 13, no. 16 (August 13, 2019): 63, DOI: 10.1186/s12966-019-0824-3, PMID: 31409357, PMCID: PMC6693254.

4. Kou Murayama et al., "When Enough Is Not Enough: Information Overload and Metacognitive Decisions to Stop Studying Information," *Journal of Experimental Psychology, Learning, Memory, and Cognition* 42, no. 6 (June 2016): 914–924, DOI: 10.1037/xlm0000213, PMCID: PMC4877291, NIHMSID: NIHMS732615, PMID: 26595067.

5. Jon Kabat-Zinn, *Mindfulness for Beginners: Reclaiming the Present Moment and Your Life* (Boulder, CO: Sounds True, 2016).

6. Edmund Husserl, *Ideas: General Introduction to Pure Phenomenology* (Mansfield Center, CT: Martino Fine Books, 2017).

7. Shian-Ling Keng, Moria J. Smoski, and Clive J. Robins, "Effects of Mindfulness on Psychological Health: A Review of Empirical Studies," *Clinical Psychology Review* 31, no. 6 (2011): 1041–1056, https://doi.org/10.1016/j.cpr.2011.04.006, PMCID: PMC3679190, NIHMSID: NIHMS463108 PMID: 21802619.

8. Sophie Middleton et al., "Factors Affecting Individual Task Prioritisation in a Workplace Setting," *Future Healthcare Journal* 5, no. 2 (June 2018): 138–142, https://doi.org/10.7861/futurehosp.5-2-138, PMID: 31098549, PMCID: PMC6502562.

9. Alessia Rosi et al., "The Impact of Failures and Successes on Affect and Self-Esteem in Young and Older Adults," *Frontiers in Psychology* 10 (August 6, 2019), https://doi.org/10.3389/fpsyg.2019.01795.

10. Mervin Blair et al., "The Role of Age and Inhibitory Efficiency in Working Memory Processing and Storage Components," *The Quarterly Journal of Experimental Psychology* 64, no. 6 (June 2011): 1157–1172, DOI: 10.1080/17470218.2010.540670, PMID: 21298594.

11. Laura Mandolesi et al., "Effects of Physical Exercise on Cognitive Functioning and Wellbeing: Biological and Psychological Benefits," *Frontiers in Psychology* 9 (April 27, 2018), https://doi.org/10.3389/fpsyg.2018.00509, PMCID: PMC593499, PMID: 29755380.

12. Marilyn Oppezzo and Daniel L. Schwartz, "Give Your Ideas Some Legs: The Positive Effect of Walking on Creative Thinking," *Journal of Experimental Psychology: Learning, Memory, and Cognition* 40, no. 4 (2014): 1142–1152.

13. Paul J. Lucassen et al., "Neuropathology of Stress," *Acta Neuropathologica* 127, no. 1 (2014): 109–135. DOI: 10.1007/s00401-013-1223-5, PMCID: PMC3889685, PMID: 24318124.

14. Chet C. Sherwood, Francys Subiaul, and Tadeusz W. Zawidzki, "A Natural History of the Human Mind: Tracing Evolutionary Changes in Brain and Cognition," 426–454.

15. Greta Mikneviciute et al., "Does Older Adults' Cognition Particularly Suffer from Stress? A Systematic Review of Acute Stress Effects on Cognition in Older Age," *Neuroscience & Biobehavioral Reviews* 132 (January 2022): 583–602.

16. June Kume, "Meditation and Mindfulness Peer-Reviewed Literature: Review," *Journal of Yoga and Physiotherapy* 5, no. 4 (July 17, 2018), DOI:10.19080/JYP.2018.05.555669.

17. Gaël Chételat et al., "Why Could Meditation Practice Help Promote Mental Health and Well-Being in Aging?" *Alzheimers Research Therapy* 10, no. 1 (2018): 57, DOI: 10.1186/s13195-018-0388-5, PMCID: PMC6015474, PMID: 29933746.

CHAPTER 10

1. Steve Maraboli, *Life, the Truth, and Being Free* (Port Washington, NY: Better Today Publishing, November 10, 2009).

2. Gil D. Rabinovici, MD; Melanie L. Stephens, PhD; and Katherine L. Possin, PhD, "Executive Dysfunction," *Continuum, Behavioral Neurology and Neuropsychiatry* 21, no. 3 (June 2015): 646–659, DOI: 1212/01.CON.00004666 58.05156.54, PMCID: PMC4455841, PMID: 26039846.

3. Ibid.

4. Rawan Tarawneh and David M. Holtzman, "The Clinical Problem of Symptomatic Alzheimer Disease and Mild Cognitive Impairment," *Cold Spring Harbor Perspectives in Medicine* 2, no. 5 (May 2012), DOI:10.1101/cshperspect. a006148.

5. Wei Sophia Deng and Vladimir M. Sloutsky, "The Development of Categorization: Effects of Classification and Inference Training on Category Representation," *Developmental Psychology* 51, no. 3 (2015): 392–405. DOI: 10.1037/a0038749, PMID: 25602938, PMCID: PMC4339312.

6. Phillippa Lally, Cornelia H. M. van Jaarsveld, Henry W. W. Potts, and Jan Wardle, "How Are Habits Formed: Modelling Habit Formation in the Real

World," *European Journal of Social Psychology* 40, no. 6 (July 16, 2009): 998–1009, https://doi.org/10.1002/ejsp.674.

7. Steven M. Smith, Arthur Glenberg, Robert A. Bjork, "Environmental Context and Human Memory," *Memory & Cognition* 6 (1978): 342–353, https://doi.org/10.3758/BF03197465.

8. Elizabeth J. Sander, Arran Caza, and Peter J. Jordan, "Psychological Perceptions Matter: Developing the Reactions to the Physical Work Environment Scale," *Building and Environment* 148, no. 15 (January 2019): 338–347, https://doi.org/10.1016/j.buildenv.2018.11.020.

9. Jeanne M. Sorrell, "Tidying Up: Good for the Aging Brain," *Journal of Psychosocial Nursing and Mental Health Services* 58, no. 4 (April 2020): 16–18, DOI: 10.3928/02793695-20200316-02, PMID: 32219461.

10. Marie Kondo, *The Life-Changing Magic of Tidying Up: The Japanese Art of Decluttering and Organizing* (Emeryville, CA: Ten Speed Press, 2014).

11. Daniela Vilaverde, Jorge Gonçalves, and Pedro Morgado, "Hoarding Disorder: A Case Report," *Frontiers in Psychiatry* 8 (June 28, 2017): 112, DOI: 10.3389/fpsyt.2017.00112, PMCID: PMC5487393, PMID: 28701963.

12. Ivo Todorov, Fabio Del Missier, and Timo Mäntylä, "Age-Related Differences in Multiple Task Monitoring," *PLoS One* 9, no. 9 (September 12, 2014): e107619, DOI: 10.1371/journal.pone.0107619, PMID: 25215609, PMCID: PMC4162647.

13. Hironori Ohsugi et al., "Differences in Dual-Task Performance and Prefrontal Cortex Activation Between Younger and Older Adults," *BMC Neuroscience* 14, no. 10 (January 18, 2013), https://doi.org/10.1186/1471-2202-14-10.

14. Alice Calaprice (ed), *The Ultimate Quotable Einstein* (Princeton, NJ: Princeton University Press, 2010): 482.

15. J. L. Quinn and Will Cresswell, "Predator Hunting Behaviour and Prey Vulnerability," *Journal of Animal Ecology* 73, no. 1 (2004): 143–154, https://www.jstor.org/stable/3505324.

16. Frederico Lourenco and B. J. Casey, "Adjusting Behavior to Changing Environmental Demands with Development," *Neuroscience and Biobehavorial Reviews* 37, 9, part B (2013): 2233–42, DOI: 10.1016/j.neubiorev.2013.03.003, PMID: 23518271, PMCID: PMC3751996, NIHMSID: NIHMS459426.

17. Sundeep Teki et al., "Brain Bases for Auditory Stimulus-Driven Figure—Ground Segregation," *Journal of Neuroscience* 31, no. 1 (January 5, 2011): 164–171, https://doi.org/10.1523/JNEUROSCI.3788-10.2011.

18. Janina A. M. Lehmann and Tina Seufert, "The Influence of Background Music on Learning in the Light of Different Theoretical Perspectives and the Role of Working Memory Capacity," *Frontiers in Psychology* 8 (October 31, 2017), https://doi.org/10.3389/fpsyg.2017.01902, PMCID: PMC5671572, PMID: 29163283.

19. Mohammad Javad Jafari et al., "The Effect of Noise Exposure on Cognitive Performance and Brain Activity Patterns," *Open Access Macedonian Journal*

of Medical Sciences 7, no. 17 (September 2019): 2924–2931, DOI: 10.3889/oamjms.2019.742, PMCID: PMC6901841, PMID: 31844459.

20. Martin R. Vasilev, Julie A. Kirkby, and Bernhard Angele, "Auditory Distraction During Reading: A Bayesian Meta-Analysis of a Continuing Controversy," *Perspectives on Psychological Science: A Journal of the Association for Psychological Science* 13, no. 5 (2018): 567–597, DOI: 10.1177/1745691617747398, PMID: 29958067, PMCID: PMC6139986.

21. Miriam I. Marrufo-Pérez, Almudena Eustaquio-Martín, and Enrique A. Lopez-Poveda, "Adaptation to Noise in Human Speech Recognition Unrelated to the Medial Olivocochlear Reflex," *Journal of Neuroscience* 38, no. 17 (April 25, 2018): 4138–4145, https://doi.org/10.1523/jneurosci.0024-18.2018.

22. Miriam I. Marrufo-Pérez et al., "Adaptation to Noise in Human Speech Recognition Depends on Noise-Level Statistics and Fast Dynamic-Range Compression," *Journal of Neuroscience* 40, no. 34 (August 19, 2020): 6613–6623, https://doi.org/10.1523/JNEUROSCI.0469-20.2020.

23. Stanley A. Goldberg, *Clinical Skills for Speech Language Pathologists* (San Diego, CA: Singular Publishing Group, 1997).

CHAPTER 11

1. Ulrich Boser, "Learning Is a Learned Behavior. Here's How to Get Better At It," *Harvard Business Review* (May 2018), https://hbr.org/2018/05/learning-is-a-learned-behavior-heres-how-to-get-better-at-it.

2. Fatima Lateef, "Simulation-Based Learning: Just Like the Real Thing, *Journal of Emergencies, Trauma, and Shock* 3, no. 4 (2010): 348–352, DOI: 10.4103/0974-2700.70743, PMID: 21063557, PMCID: PMC2966567.

3. Kyle Mills, "The 10 Secrets of Success by Bob Bowman," *American Swimming Coaches Association* (January 2017).

4. Eleanor A. Maguire et al., "Navigation-Related Structural Change in the Hippocampi of Taxi Drivers," *PNAS* 97, no. 8 (2000): 4398–4403; https://doi.org/10.1073/pnas.070039597.

5. Phillippa Lally et al., "How Are Habits Formed: Modelling Habit Formation in the Real World," *European Journal of Social Psychology* 40, no. 6 (July 16, 2009): 998–1009, https://doi.org/10.1002/ejsp.674.

6. William Epstein and Barbara E. Lovitts, "Automatic and Attentional Components in Perception of Shape-at-a-Slant," *Journal of Experimental Psychology: Human Perception and Performance* 11, no. 3 (1985): 355–366, https://doi.org/10.1037/0096-1523.11.3.355.

7. Karen D. Ersche et al., "Creature of Habit: A Self-Report Measure of Habitual Routines and Automatic Tendencies in Everyday Life," *Personality and Individual Differences* 116 (October 2017): 73–85, https://doi.org/10.1016/j.paid.2017.04.024, PMCID: PMC5473478 PMID: 28974825.

8. "Daily Routines and Habits of Famous Musicians," *Cardon Studios*, (October 8, 2015), https://cardonstudios.com/daily-routines-and-habits-of-famous-musicians.

9. Mathieu Servant et al., "Neural Bases of Automaticity," *Journal of Experimental Psychology, Learning, Memory, and Cognition* 44, no. 3 (2018): 440–464, DOI: 10.1037/xlm0000454, PMCID: PMC5862722, NIHMSID: NIHMS894496, PMID: 28933906.

10. C. S. Green and D. Bavelier, "Exercising Your Brain: A Review of Human Brain Plasticity and Training-Induced Learning," *Psychology and Aging* 23, no. 4 (December 2008): 692–701. DOI: 10.1037/a0014345, PMID: 19140641, PMCID: PMC2896818.

11. Mark P. Mattson, "Superior Pattern Processing is the Essence of the Evolved Human Brain," *Frontiers in Neuroscience* 8 (August 22, 2014): 265, https://doi.org/10.3389/fnins.2014.00265, PMCID: PMC4141622, PMID: 25202234.

12. Jeremy E. Sherman, PhD, "Psychological Crutches: Ten Myths and Three Tips," *Psychology Today* (April 17, 2014), https://www.psychologytoday.com/us/blog/ambigamy/201404/psychological-crutches-ten-myths-and-three-tips.

13. John Lisman, "The Challenge of Understanding the Brain: Where We Stand in 2015," *Neuron* 86, no. 4 (May 2015): 864–882, DOI: 10.1016/j.neuron.2015.03.032, PMID: 25996132, PMCID: PMC4441769.

Chapter 12

1. Janet Metcalfe, "Learning from Errors," *Annual Review of Psychology* 68, no. 1 (2017): 465–489.

2. Leonid Perlovsky, "A Challenge to Human Evolution-Cognitive Dissonance," *Frontiers in Psychology* 4 (April 10, 2013):179, DOI: 10.3389/fpsyg.2013.00179, PMID: 23596433, PMCID: PMC3622034.

3. Saul Mcleod, "What Is Cognitive Dissonance? Definition and Examples," *Simply Psychology* (March 6, 2023).

4. Ralf C. Buckley, "Aging Adventure Athletes Assess Achievements and Alter Aspirations to Maintain Self-Esteem," *Frontiers in Psychology* 9 (2018): 225, https://doi.org/10.3389/fpsyg.2018.00225.

5. Kevin Lane Keller, "Consumer Research Insights on Brands and Branding: A JCR Curation," *Journal of Consumer Research* 46, no. 5 (2020): 995–1001, https://doi.org/10.1093/jcr/ucz058.

6. Peter Gärdenfors, *Conceptual Spaces: The Geometry of Thought* (Cambridge, MA: MIT Press/Bradford Books, 2004).

7. Bettina Höchli, Adrian Brügger, and Claude Messner, "How Focusing on Superordinate Goals Motivates Broad, Long-Term Goal Pursuit: A Theoretical Perspective," *Frontiers in Psychology* 9 (2018): 1879, https://doi.org/10.3389/fpsyg.2018.01879, PMCID: PMC6176065, PMID: 30333781.

CHAPTER 13

1. William Shakespeare, *Macbeth* (Wordsworth Classics, 1992).

2. Claire E. Sexton et al., "Poor Sleep Quality is Associated with Increased Cortical Atrophy in Community-Dwelling Adults," *Neurology* 83, no. 11 (September 9, 2014): 967–973, https://doi.org/10.1212/WNL.0000000000000774.

3. Kendra Cherry, "The 4 Stages of Sleep: What Happens in the Brain and Body During NREM and REM Sleep," VeryWellHealth (October 2, 2022), https://www.verywellhealth.com/the-four-stages-of-sleep-2795920.

4. Susan L. Worley, "The Extraordinary Importance of Sleep: The Detrimental Effects of Inadequate Sleep on Health and Public Safety Drive an Explosion of Sleep Research," *Pharmacy and Therapeutics* 43, no. 12 (December 2018): 758–763, PMID: 30559589, PMCID: PMC6281147.

5. E. Shokri-Kojori et al., "ß-Amyloid Accumulation in the Human Brain After One Night of Sleep Deprivation," *Proceedings of the National Academy of Sciences* (PNAS) 115, no. 17, (April 9, 2018): 4483–4488, https://doi.org/10.1073/pnas.1721694115, PMID: 29632177.

6. Björn Rash and Jan Born, "About Sleep's Role in Memory," *Physiological Reviews* 93, no. 2 (2013): 681–766, DOI: 10.1152/physrev.00032.2012, PMCID: PMC3768102, PMID: 23589831.

7. Ibid.

8. Paula Alhola and Päivi Polo-Kantola, "Sleep Deprivation: Impact on Cognitive Performance," *Neuropsychiatric Disease and Treatment* 3, no. 5 (October 2007): 553–567, PMCID: PMC2656292, PMID: 19300585.

9. Jean-Philippe Chaput, Caroline Dutil, and Hugues Sampasa-Kanyinga, "Sleeping Hours: What Is the Ideal Number and How Does Age Impact This?" *Nature and Science of Sleep* 10 (2018): 421–430, DOI: 10.2147/NSS.S163071, PMCID: PMC6267703, PMID: 30568521.

10. Adrianna Huffington, *The Sleep Revolution* (New York: Harmony, 2016).

11. J. F. Pagel, Bennett L. Parnes, "Medications for the Treatment of Sleep Disorders: An Overview," *Primary Care Companion to the Journal of Clinical Psychiatry* 3, no. 3 (2001): 118–125, DOI: 10.4088/pcc.v03n0303, PMID: 15014609, PMCID: PMC181172.

12. Kirstie N. Anderson, "Insomnia and Cognitive Behavioural Therapy—How to Assess Your Patient and Why It Should Be a Standard Part of Care," *Journal of Thoracic Disease* 10, no. 1 (2018): S94–S102, DOI: 10.21037/jtd.2018.01.35, PMID: 29445533, PMCID: PMC5803038.

13. Kazue Okamoto-Mizuno and Koh Mizuno, "Effects of Thermal Environment on Sleep and Circadian Rhythm," *Journal of Physiological Anthropology* 31, no. 14 (2012), https://doi.org/10.1186/1880-6805-31-14, PMID: 22738673, PMCID: PMC3427038.

14. Ibid.

15. Danielle Pacheco, "The Best Temperature for Sleep," The Sleep Foundation (September 29, 2022), https://www.sleepfoundation.org/bedroom-environment

/best-temperature-for-sleep#:~:text=A%20National%20Sleep%20Foundation %20poll,Fahrenheit%20(18.3%20degrees%20Celsius).

16. Demian Halperin, "Environmental Noise and Sleep Disturbances: A Threat to Health?" *Sleep Science* 7, no 4 (2014): 209–212, DOI: 10.1016/j. slsci.2014.11.003, PMID: 26483931, PMCID: PMC4608916.

17. Christine Blume, Corrado Garbazza, Manuel Spitschan, "Effects of Light on Human Circadian Rhythms, Sleep and Mood," *Somnologie (Berlin)* 23, no. 3 (August 19, 2019): 147–156, DOI: 10.1007/s11818-019-00215-x, PMID: 31534436, PMCID: PMC6751071.

18. Goran Medic, Micheline Wille, Michiel Eh Hemels, "Short- and Long-Term Health Consequences of Sleep Disruption," *Nature and Science of Sleep* 19, no. 9 (2017): 151–161, https://doi.org/10.2147/NSS.S134864, PMID: 28579842, PMCID: PMC5449130.

19. Eve Van Cauter et al., "Nocturnal Decrease in Glucose Tolerance During Constant Glucose Infusion," *Journal of Clinical Endocrinology & Metabolism* 69, no. 3 (1989): 604–611, https://doi.org/10.1210/jcem-69-3-604.

20. Amber W. Kinsey and Michael J. Ormsbee, "The Health Impact of Nighttime Eating: Old and New Perspectives," *Nutrients* 7, no. 4 (2015): 2648– 2662, DOI: https://doi.org/10.3390/nu7042648, PMID: 25859885, PMCID: PMC4425165.

21. N Chung, Y. S. Bin, P.A. Cistulli and C.M. Chow. "Does the Proximity of Meals to Bedtime Influence the Sleep of Young Adults? A Cross-Sectional Survey of University Students. *Int J Environ Res Public Health.* 2020 Apr 14;17(8):2677. doi: 10.3390/ijerph17082677. PMID: 32295235; PMCID: PMC7215804.

22. Julia Pietilä et al., "Acute Effect of Alcohol Intake on Cardiovascular Autonomic Regulation During the First Hours of Sleep in a Large Real-World Sample of Finnish Employees: Observational Study," *JMIR Mental Health.* 16; 5, no. (1) (Mar 2018):e23., https://doi.org/10.2196/mental.9519, DOI: 10.2196/ mental.9519. PMID: 29549064;, PMCID: PMC5878366.

23. Soon-Yeob Park et al., "The Effects of Alcohol on Quality of Sleep," *Korean Journal of Family Medicine* 36, no. 6 (2015): 294–9, https://doi.org/10 .4082/kjfm.2015.36.6.294, PMID: 26634095; PMCID: PMC4666864.

24. Gianluca Tosini, Ian Ferguson, and Kazuo Tsubota, "Effects of Blue Light on the Circadian System and Eye Physiology," *Molecular Vision* 22 (2016): 61–72, PMID: 26900325, PMCID: PMC4734149.

25. Ari Shechter et al., "Blocking Nocturnal Blue Light for Insomnia: A Randomized Controlled Trial," *Journal of Psychiatric Research* 96 (2018): 196–202, DOI: 10.1016/j.jpsychires.2017.10.015, PMID: 29101797, PMCID: PMC5703049.

26. Arianna Huffington, *The Sleep Revolution* (New York, NY: Harmony, 2016).

27. Carl Sagan, *Cosmos* (New York, NY: Random House, 1983).

28. Brett A. Dolezal et al., "Interrelationship Between Sleep and Exercise: A Systematic Review," *Advances in Preventive Medicine* (2017), https://doi.org/10.1155/2017/1364387, PMID: 28458924, PMCID: PMC5385214.

29. Johns Hopkins Hospital, "Exercising for Better Sleep," (November 18, 2022), https://www.hopkinsmedicine.org/health/wellness-and-prevention/exercising-for-better-sleep.

30. Dolezal, "Interrelationship between Sleep and Exercise: A Systematic Review."

31. Diva Parekh, "Learning to Listen to My Mind and My Body," *Johns Hopkins News-Letter* (January 30, 2020).

32. Frédéric Dutheil et al., "Effects of a Short Daytime Nap on the Cognitive Performance: A Systematic Review and Meta-Analysis," *International Journal of Environmental Research and Public Health* 18, no. 19 (2021), https://doi.org/10.3390/ijerph181910212, PMID: 34639511, PMCID: PMC8507757.

CHAPTER 14

1. Fernando Gómez-Pinilla, "Brain Foods: The Effects of Nutrients on Brain Function," *Nature Reviews Neuroscience* 9, no. 7 (July 2008): 568–578, https://doi.org/10.1038/nrn2421, PMID: 18568016, PMCID: PMC2805706.

2. Sanjay Gupta, *Keep Sharp: Build a Better Brain at Any Age* (New York: Simon & Shuster, 2021).

3. Jianfen Zhang et al., "The Effects of Hydration Status on Cognitive Performances Among Young Adults in Hebei, China: A Randomized Controlled Trial (RCT)," *International Journal of Environmental Research and Public Health* 15, no. 7 (July 2018): 1477, https://doi.org/10.3390/ijerph15071477, PMCID: PMC6068860 PMID: 30720789.

4. Barry M. Popkin, Kristen E. D'Anci, Irwin H. Rosenberg, "Water, Hydration, and Health," *Nutrition Reviews* 68, no. 8 (August 2010): 439–458, https://doi.org/10.1111/j.1753-4887.2010.00304.x, PMID: 20646222, PMCID: PMC2908954.

5. Gómez-Pinilla, "Brain Foods: The Effects of Nutrients on Brain Function," 568–578.

6. Joyce C. McCann and Bruce N. Ames, "Is Docosahexaenoic Acid, an N-3 Long-Chain Polyunsaturated Fatty Acid, Required for Development of Normal Brain Function? An Overview of Evidence from Cognitive and Behavioral Tests in Humans and Animals," *American Journal of Clinical Nutrition* 82, no. 2 (2005):281–295, https://doi.org/10.1093/ajcn.82.2.281, PMID: 16087970.

7. Carol E. Greenwood and Gordon Winocur, "High-Fat Diets, Insulin Resistance and Declining Cognitive Function," *Neurobiology of Aging* 26, no. 1 (2005): 42–45, https://doi.org/10.1016/j.neurobiolaging.2005.08.017, PMID: 16257476.

8. S. A. Frautschy et al. "Phenolic Anti-Inflammatory Antioxidant Reversal of a Aß-Induced Cognitive Deficits and Neuropathology," *Neurobiology of Aging* 22, no. 6 (2001): 993–1005, https://doi.org/10.1016/S0197-4580(01)00300-1.

9. L. Letenneur et al., "Flavonoid Intake and Cognitive Decline Over a 10-Year Period," *American Journal of Epidemiology* 165, no. 12 (2007): 1364–1371, https://doi.org/10.1093/aje/kwm036.

10. Janet Bryan, Eva Calvaresi, and Donna Hughes, "Short-Term Folate, Vitamin B-12 or Vitamin B-6 Supplementation Slightly Affects Memory Performance but Not Mood in Women of Various Ages," *Journal of Nutrition* 132, no. 6 (2002): 1345–1356, https://doi.org/10.1093/jn/132.6.1345.

11. Nikolaj Travica et al., "Vitamin C Status and Cognitive Function: A Systematic Review," *Nutrients* 9, no. 9 (August 2017): 960, https://doi.org/10.3390/nu9090960, PMID: 28867798, PMCID: PMC5622720.

12. Robert J. Przybelski and Neil C. Binkley, "Is Vitamin D Important for Preserving Cognition? A Positive Correlation of Serum 25-Hydroxyvitamin D Concentration with Cognitive Function," *Archives of Biochemistry and Biophysics* 460, no. 2 (2007): 202–205, https://doi.org/10.1016/j.abb.2006.12.018.

13. Anthony J. Perkins et al. "Association of Antioxidants with Memory in a Multiethnic Elderly Sample Using the Third National Health and Nutrition Examination Survey," *American Journal of Epidemiology* 150, no. 1, (1999): 37–44, https://doi.org/10.1093/oxfordjournals.aje.a009915.

14. M. Fava et al., "Folate, Vitamin B12, and Homocysteine in Major Depressive Disorder," *American Journal of Psychiatry* 154, no. 3 (1997): 426–428, https://doi.org/10.1176/ajp.154.3.426.

15. James A. Joseph, Barbara Shukitt-Hale, Francis C. Lau, "Fruit Polyphenols and Their Effects on Neuronal Signaling and Behavior in Senescence," *Annals of the New York Academy of Sciences* 1100 (2007): 470–485, https://doi.org/10.1196/annals.1395.052.

16. Greenwood, "High-Fat Diets, Insulin Resistance and Declining Cognitive Function," 42–45.

17. C. P. Chong et al., "Habitual Sugar Intake and Cognitive Impairment Among Multi-Ethnic Malaysian Older Adults," *Clinical Interventions in Aging* 14 (July 2019): 1331–1342, https://doi.org/10.2147/CIA.S211534, PMID: 31413554, PMCID: PMC6662517.

18. Keith E. Pearson et al., "Dietary Patterns Are Associated with Cognitive Function in the Reasons for Geographic and Racial Differences in Stroke (REGARDS) Cohort," *Journal of Nutritional Science* 5, no. 38 (2016), https://doi.org/10.1017/jns.2016.27, PMID: 27752305, PMCID: PMC5048188.

19. James E. Gangwisch et al., "High Glycemic Index Diet as a Risk Factor for Depression: Analyses from the Women's Health Initiative," *American Journal of Clinical Nutrition* 102, no. 2 (August 2015): 454–463, https://doi.org/10.3945/ajcn.114.103846, PMID: 26109579, PMCID: PMC4515860.

20. Seva G. Khambadkone et al., "Nitrated Meat Products are Associated with Mania in Humans and Altered Behavior and Brain Gene Expression in Rats," *Molecular Psychiatry* 25, no. 3 (March 2020): 560–571, https://doi.org/10.1038/s41380-018-0105-6, PMID: 30022042, PMCID: PMC7077736.

CHAPTER 15

1. Donald Rumsfeld's response to a question at a U.S. Department of Defense news briefing on February 12, 2002.

2. Note: People use the words "dementia" and "Alzheimer's" interchangeably. However, Alzheimer's is only one of the many forms of dementia. When I use "dementia" in the book, it includes Alzheimer's.

3. Luís Felipe José Ravic de Miranda et al., "Factors Influencing Possible Delay in the Diagnosis of Alzheimer's Disease: Findings from a Tertiary Public University Hospital," *Dementia & Neuropsychologia* 5, no. 4 (2011): 328–331, https://doi.org/10.1590/S1980-57642011DN05040011, PMCID: PMC5619046, PMID: 29213760.

4. Zachariah M. Reagh et al., "Functional Imbalance of Anterolateral Entorhinal Cortex and Hippocampal Dentate/CA3 Underlies Age-Related Object Pattern Separation Deficits," *Neuron* 97, no. 5 (March 2018): 1187–1198, https://doi.org/10.1016/j.neuron.2018.01.039, PMID: 29518359, PMCID: PMC5937538.

5. Dalai Lama, *The Universe in a Single Atom: The Convergence of Science and Spirituality* (New York: Harmony, 2006).

6. Ruth Bader Ginsburg, *Dissent on Gonzales v. Carhart*, 05–380 F.3d 791, 05–1382 435 F. 3d 1163, reversed (Supreme Court of the United States).

7. Richard P. Feynman, *The Pleasure of Finding Things Out: The Best Short Works of Richard P. Feynman* (Long Island City, NY: Helix Books, 1999).

8. Abubaker Elbayoudi et al., "Trend Analysis Techniques in Forecasting Human Behaviour Evolution," *PETRA '17: Proceedings of the 10th International Conference on Pervasive Technologies Related to Assistive Environments* (June 2017): 293–299, https://doi.org/10.1145/3056540.3076198.

9. James A. Wilcox and Reid Duffy, "Is It a 'Senior Moment' or Early Dementia? Addressing Memory Concerns in Older Patients," *Current Psychiatry* 15, no. 5 (May 2016): 28–30, 32–34, 40.

10. Abhilash K. Desai, "Subjective Cognitive Impairment: When to Be Concerned About 'Senior Moments,'" *Current Psychiatry* 10, no. 4 (April 2011): 31–45.

11. Stanley A. Goldberg, *Clinical Skills for Speech-Language Pathologists* (San Diego: Singular Publishing, 1997).

12. Vaisakh Puthusseryppady et al., "Spatial Disorientation in Alzheimer's Disease: The Missing Path from Virtual Reality to Real World," *Frontiers in Aging Neuroscience* 12 (October 27, 2020), https://doi.org/10.3389/fnagi.2020.550514, PMID: 33192453, PMCID: PMC7652847.

13. Stan Goldberg, *Leaning into Sharp Points: Practical Guidance and Nurturing Support for Caregivers* (Novato: New World Library, 2012).

14. Daniel C. Mograbi, Robin G. Morris, "Anosognosia," *Cortex: A Journal Devoted to the Study of the Nervous System and Behavior* 103 (June 2018): 385–386, https://doi.org/10.1016/j.cortex.2018.04.001, PMID: 29731103.

15. Joseph Therriault et al., "Anosognosia Predicts Default Mode Network Hypometabolism and Clinical Progression to Dementia," *Neurology* 90, no. 11 (2018), https://doi.org/10.1212/WNL.0000000000005120, PMID: 29444971, PMCID: PMC5858945.

16. National Institutes of Health, "Alzheimer's Disease" (2018), https://www.nih.gov/research-training/accelerating-medicines-partnership-amp/alzheimers-disease.

17. Kimberly Holland, "Life Expectancy and Long-Term Outlook for Alzheimer's Disease," *Healthline* (September 29, 2018), https://www.healthline.com/health/alzheimers-disease/life-expectancy.

18. René J. F. Melis, Miriam L. Haaksma, Graciela Muniz-Terrera, "Understanding and Predicting the Longitudinal Course of Dementia," *Current Opinion in Psychiatry* 32, no. 2 (2019): 123–129, https://doi.org/10.1097/YCO.0000000000000482, PMCID: PMC6380437, PMID: 30557268.

19. Allan B. Schwarz, "Medical Mystery: Did Reagan have Alzheimer's While President?" *Philadelphia Inquirer* (August 13, 2016).

20. Stanley A. Goldberg, *Ready to Learn: How to Help Your Preschooler Succeed.* (New York: Oxford University Press, 2005).

21. R. Robinson, "Cost-Benefit Analysis," *BMJ* 307, no. 6909 (October 1993): 924–926, https://doi.org/10.1136/bmj.307.6909.924, PMCID: PMC1679054, PMID: 8241859.

22. Richard J. Kryscio et al., "Self-Reported Memory Complaints: Implications from a Longitudinal Cohort with Autopsies," *Neurology* 83, no. 15 (September 2014): 1359–1365, https://doi.org/10.1212/WNL.0000000000000856, PMID: 25253756, PMCID: PMC4189103.

BIBLIOGRAPHY

"A Day in the Life: Stephen Curry." *Owaves* (June 12, 2018). https://owaves
  .com/day-plans/day-life-stephen-curry.
Adolphs, Ralph. "The Social Brain: Neural Basis of Social Knowledge." *Annual
  Review Psychology* 60 (January 10, 2009): 693–716. DOI: 10.1146/annurev.
  psych.60.110707.163514, PMID: 18771388, PMCID: PMC2588649.
Afaghi, A., Helen O'Connor, and Chin Moi Chow. "High-Glycemic-Index
  Carbohydrate Meals Shorten Sleep Onset." *American Journal of Clinical
  Nutrition* 85, no. 2. (2007): 426–430. https://doi.org/10.1093/ajcn/85.2
  .426.
Alhola, Paula, and Päivi Polo-Kantola. "Sleep Deprivation: Impact on Cognitive
  Performance." *Neuropsychiatric Disease and Treatment* 3, no. 5 (October
  2007): 553–567. PMCID: PMC2656292, PMID: 19300585.
Anderson, Kirstie N. "Insomnia and Cognitive Behavioural Therapy—How
  to Assess Your Patient and Why It Should Be a Standard Part of Care."
  Journal of Thoracic Disease 10, no. 1 (2018): S94–S102. DOI: 10.21037/
  jtd.2018.01.35, PMID: 29445533, PMCID: PMC5803038.
Atkinson, Jaye L. "Senior Moments: The Acceptability of an Ageist Phrase."
  Journal of Aging Studies 18, no. 2 (May 2004): 123–142. DOI: 10.1016/j.
  jaging.2004.01.008.
Baddeley, Alan. "Working Memory: Theories, Models, and Controversies."
  Annual Review of Psychology 63 (2012): 1–29. https://doi.org/10.1146/
  annurev-psych-120710-100422.
Bature, Fidelia, Barbara-ann Guinn, Dong Pang, and Yannis Pappas. "Signs and
  Symptoms Preceding the Diagnosis of Alzheimer's Disease: A Systematic
  Scoping Review of Literature from 1937 to 2016." *BMJ Open* 7, no. 8
  (August 28, 2017). https://doi.org/10.1136/bmjopen-2016-015746.
The Beach Boys, *Surfin' Safari*, Capital, 1962.
Berlin, Isaiah. *The Proper Study of Mankind: An Anthology of Essays* (New York,
  NY: Farrar, Straus, and Giroux, 2000).
Berra, Yogi. *The Yogi Book*. New York City: Workingman Publishing, 2010.
Bishop, Nicholas A., Tao Lu, and Bruce A. Yankner. "Neural Mechanisms
  of Ageing and Cognitive Decline." *Nature* 464, no. 7288 (March

2010): 529–35. DOI: 10.1038/nature08983, PMID: 20336135, PMCID: PMC2927852.

Blair, Mervin, Kiran K. Vadaga, Joni Shuchat, and Karen Z. H. Li. "The Role of Age and Inhibitory Efficiency in Working Memory Processing and Storage Components." *The Quarterly Journal of Experimental Psychology* 64, no. 6 (June 2011): 1157–1172. DOI: 10.1080/17470218.2010.540670, PMID: 21298594.

Blasche, Gerhard, Barbara Szabo, Michaela Wagner-Menghin, Cem Ekmekcioglu, and Erwin Gollner. "Comparison of Rest-Break Interventions During a Mentally Demanding Task." *Stress Health* 34, no. 5 (2018): 629–638. https://doi.org/10.1002/smi.2830, PMID: 30113771, PMCID: PMC6585675.

Blume, Christine, Corrado Garbazza, and Manuel Spitschan. "Effects of Light on Human Circadian Rhythms, Sleep and Mood." *Somnologie (Berlin)* 23, no. 3 (August 19, 2019): 147–156. DOI: 10.1007/s11818-019-00215-x, PMID: 31534436, PMCID: PMC6751071.

Boser, Ulrich. "Learning Is a Learned Behavior. Here's How to Get Better at It." *Harvard Business Review* (May 2018). https://hbr.org/2018/05/learning-is-a-learned-behavior-heres-how-to-get-better-at-it.

Bosker, Hans Rutger, David Peeters, and Judith Holler. "How Visual Cues to Speech Rate Influence Speech Perception." *Quarterly Journal of Experimental Psychology* 73, no. 10 (2020): 1523–1536. https://doi.org/10.1177/1747021820914564.

Bouton, Mark E. "Why Behavior Change is Difficult to Sustain." *Preventive Medicine* 68 (November 2014): 29–36. https://doi.org/10.1016/j.ypmed.2014.06.010, PMCID: PMC4287360, NIHMSID: NIHMS605603, PMID: 24937649.

Berry, Brandon. "Minimizing Confusion and Disorientation: Cognitive Support Work in Informal Dementia Caregiving." *Journal of Aging Studies* 30 (2014): 121–130. DOI: 10.1016/j.jaging.2014.05.001, PMCID: PMC4443911, NIHMSID: NIHMS594723, PMID: 24984915.

Bridge, Donna J., and Ken A. Paller. "Neural Correlates of Reactivation and Retrieval-Induced Distortion." *Journal of Neuroscience* 32, no. 35 (2012): 12144–12151. DOI: 10.1523/jneurosci.1378-12.2012.

Brilliant T., Denilson, Rui Nouchi, and Ryuta Kawashima. "Does Video Gaming Have Impacts on the Brain: Evidence from a Systematic Review." *Brain Sciences* 9, no. 10 (September 2019): 251. DOI: 10.3390/brainsci9100251, PMID: 31557907, PMCID: PMC6826942.

Bryan, Janet, Eva Calvaresi, and Donna Hughes. "Short-Term Folate, Vitamin B-12 or Vitamin B-6 Supplementation Slightly Affects Memory Performance but Not Mood in Women of Various Ages." *Journal of Nutrition* 132, no. 6 (2002): 1345–1356. https://doi.org/10.1093/jn/132.6.1345.

Buckley, Ralf C. "Aging Adventure Athletes Assess Achievements and Alter Aspirations to Maintain Self-Esteem." *Frontiers in Psychology* 9 (February 28, 2018): 225. DOI: 10.3389/fpsyg.2018.00225.

Calaprice, Alice (ed). *The Ultimate Quotable Einstein* (Princeton, NJ: Princeton University Press, 2010): 482.

Carlin, George. *Brain Droppings.* New York: Hyperion, 1998.

Cascella, Marco, and Yasir Al Khalili. *Short Term Memory Impairment* (St. Petersburg, FL: StatPearls Publishing, 2022).

Castel, Alan D. "Aging and Memory for Numerical Information: The Role of Specificity and Expertise in Associative Memory." *The Journals of Gerontology: Series B,* 62, no. 3 (May 2007): P194–P196. https://doi.org/10.1093/geronb/62.3.P194.

Chaput, Jean-Philippe, Caroline Dutil, and Hugues Sampasa-Kanyinga. "Sleeping Hours: What Is the Ideal Number and How Does Age Impact This?" *Nature and Science of Sleep* 10 (2018): 421–430. DOI: 10.2147/NSS. S163071, PMCID: PMC6267703, PMID: 30568521.

Cherry, Kendra. "The 4 Stages of Sleep: What Happens in the Brain and Body During NREM and REM Sleep." VeryWellHealth (October 2, 2022). https://www.verywellhealth.com/the-four-stages-of-sleep-2795920.

Chételat, Gaël, Antoine Lutz, Eider Arenaza-Urquijo, Fabienne Collette, Olga Klimecki, Natalie Marchant. "Why Could Meditation Practice Help Promote Mental Health and Well-Being in Aging?" *Alzheimers Research Therapy* 10, no. 1 (2018): 57. DOI: 10.1186/s13195-018-0388-5, PMCID: PMC6015474, PMID: 29933746.

Childs, Emma and Harriet de Wit. "Regular Exercise Is Associated With Emotional Resilience to Acute Stress in Healthy Adults." *Frontiers in Physiology* (May 2014): 161. DOI:10.3389/fphys.2014.00161, PMID: 24822048, PMCID: PMC4013452.

Chong, C. P., S. Shahar, H. Haron, and N. C. Din. "Habitual Sugar Intake and Cognitive Impairment Among Multi-Ethnic Malaysian Older Adults." *Clinical Interventions in Aging* 14 (July 2019): 1331–1342. https://doi.org/10.2147/CIA.S211534, PMID: 31413554, PMCID: PMC6662517.

Chung, Nikola, Yu Sun Bin, Peter A. Cistull, and Chin Moi Chow. "Does the Proximity of Meals to Bedtime Influence the Sleep of Young Adults? A Cross-Sectional Survey of University Students." *International Journal of Environmental Research and Public Health* 17, no 8. (April 14, 2020): 2677. DOI:10.3390/ijerph17082677, PMID: 32295235, PMCID: PMC7215804.

Coelho, Paulo. *The Devil and Miss Prym* (New York: Harper One, 2021).

Compernolle, Sofie, Ann DeSmet, Loise Poppe, Geert Crombez, Ilse De Bourdeaudhuij, Greet Cardon, Hidde P. van der Ploeg, Delfien Van Dyke. "Effectiveness of Interventions Using Self-Monitoring to Reduce Sedentary Behavior in Adults: A Systematic Review and Meta-Analysis."

International Journal of Behavioral Nutrition and Physical Activity 13, no. 16 (August 13, 2019): 63. DOI: 10.1186/s12966-019-0824-3, PMID: 31409357, PMCID: PMC6693254.

Cotterill, Stewart. "Preparing for Performance: Strategies Adopted Across Performance Domains." *Sport Psychologist* 29, no. 2 (2015): 158–170. https://doi.org/10.1123/tsp.2014-0035.

Cowan, Nelson. "What Are the Differences Between Long-Term, Short-Term, and Working Memory?" *Progress in Brain Research* 169 (2008): 323–338. DOI: 10.1016/S0079-6123(07)00020-9, PMCID: PMC2657600, NIHMSID: NIHMS84208, PMID: 18394484.

Craik, Fergus I. M. "Effects of Distraction on Memory and Cognition: A Commentary." *Frontiers in Psychology* 5 (2014): 841. https://doi.org/10.3389/fpsyg.2014.00841.

"Daily Routines and Habits of Famous Musicians." *Cardon Studios* (October 8, 2015). https://cardonstudios.com/daily-routines-and-habits-of-famous-musicians.

Dalai Lama. "In Praise of Dependent Arising—First Day." October 9, 2021. webcast, https://www.dalailama.com/news/2021/in-praise-of-dependent-arising-first-day.

———. The Universe in a Single Atom: The Convergence of Science and Spirituality (New York: Harmony, 2006).

De Beni, Rossana, Erika Borella, and Barbara Carretti. "Reading Comprehension in Aging: The Role of Working Memory and Metacomprehension." *Aging, Neuropsychology, and Cognition* 14, no. 2 (2007): 189–212. DOI: 10.1080/13825580500229213.

De Miranda, Luís Felipe José Ravic, Rafael de Oliveira Matoso, Marlon Viera Rodrigues, Thiago Oliveira Lemos de Lima, Adriano Fiorini Nascimento, Fernando Castro Carvalho, Debora Regina de Melo Moreira, Jeferson Cruz Fernandes, Jonas Jardi de Paula, Luiz Alexandre V. Magno, Paulo Caramelli, Edgar Nunes de Moraes. "Factors Influencing Possible Delay in the Diagnosis of Alzheimer's Disease: Findings from a Tertiary Public University Hospital." *Dementia & Neuropsychologia* 5, no. 4 (2011): 328–331. https://doi.org/10.1590/S1980-57642011DN05040011, PMCID: PMC5619046, PMID: 29213760.

Deffenbacher, Jerry L., and Richard M. Suinn. "Systematic Desensitization and the Reduction of Anxiety." *The Counseling Psychologist* 16, no. 1 (June 30, 2016). https://doi.org/10.1177/0011000088161002.

Deng, Wei Sophia, and Vladimir M. Sloutsky. "The Development of Categorization: Effects of Classification and Inference Training on Category Representation." *Developmental Psychology* 51, no. 3 (2015): 392–405. DOI: 10.1037/a0038749, PMID: 25602938, PMCID: PMC4339312.

Desai, Abhilash K. "Subjective Cognitive Impairment: When to Be Concerned About 'Senior Moments,'" *Current Psychiatry* 10, no. 4 (April 2011): 31–45.

Devitt, Aleea L., and Daniel L. Schacter. "False Memories with Age: Neural and Cognitive Underpinnings." *Neuropsychologia* 91 (October 2016): 346–359. DOI: 10.1016/j.neuropsychologia.2016.08.030, PMCID: PMC5075259, NIHMSID: NIHMS815717, PMID: 27592332.

Diamond, B. J., J. DeLuca, D. Rosenthal, R. Vlad, K. Davis, G. Lucas, O. Noskin, and J. A. Richards. "Information Processing in Older Versus Younger Adults: Accuracy Versus Speed." *International Journal of Rehabilitation and Health* 5 (2000): 55–64. https://doi.org/10.1023/A:1012911203468.

Disney, Walt. *The Way to Get Started is to Quit Talking and Begin Doing.* Independently Published, 2022.

Dolezal, Brett A., Eric V. Neufeld, David M. Boland, Jennifer L. Martin, and Christopher B. Cooper. "Interrelationship Between Sleep and Exercise: A Systematic Review." *Advances in Preventive Medicine* (2017). https://doi.org/10.1155/2017/1364387, PMID: 28458924, PMCID: PMC5385214.

Dudukovic, Nicole M., Elizabeth J. Marsh, and Barbara Tversky. "Telling a Story or Telling it Straight: The Effects of Entertaining Versus Accurate Retellings on Memory." *Applied Cognitive Psychology* 18, no 2 (2004): 125–143.

Dutheil, Frédéric, Benjamin Danini, Reza Bagheri, Maria Livia Fantini, Bruno Pereira, Farès Moustafa, Marion Trousselard, and Valentin Navel. "Effects of a Short Daytime Nap on the Cognitive Performance: A Systematic Review and Meta-Analysis." *International Journal of Environmental Research and Public Health* 18, no. 19 (2021). https://doi.org/10.3390/ijerph181910212, PMID: 34639511, PMCID: PMC8507757.

Eichenbaum, Howard. *The Cognitive Neuroscience of Memory* (New York: Oxford University Press, 2002).

Elbayoudi, Abubaker, Ahmad Lotfi, Caroline Langensiepen, Kofi Appiah. "Trend Analysis Techniques in Forecasting Human Behaviour Evolution." *PETRA '17: Proceedings of the 10th International Conference on Pervasive Technologies Related to Assistive Environments* (June 2017): 293–299. https://doi.org/10.1145/3056540.3076198.

Epstein, William, and Barbara E. Lovitts. "Automatic and Attentional Components in Perception of Shape-at-a-Slant." *Journal of Experimental Psychology: Human Perception and Performance* 11, no. 3 (1985): 355–366. https://doi.org/10.1037/0096-1523.11.3.355.

Ersche, Karen D., Tsen-Vei Lim, Laetitia H. E. Ward, Trevor W. Robbins, and Jan Stochl. "Creature of Habit: A Self-Report Measure of Habitual Routines and Automatic Tendencies in Everyday Life." *Personality and Individual Differences* 116 (October 2017): 73–85. https://doi.org/10.1016/j.paid.2017.04.024, PMCID: PMC5473478 PMID: 28974825.

Fancher, Justine Marie. "How is Comprehension Affected When Reading Aloud Versus Reading Silently?" Education and Human Development Master's Theses (2008): 276.

Fava, M., J. S. Borus, J. E. Alpert, A. A. Nierenberg, J. F. Rosenbaum, and T. Bottiglieri. "Folate, Vitamin B12, and Homocysteine in Major Depressive Disorder." *American Journal of Psychiatry* 154, no. 3 (1997): 426–428. https://doi.org/10.1176/ajp.154.3.426.

Ferrari, Joseph R., Juan Francisco Díaz-Morales, Jean O'Callaghan, Karem Díaz, and Doris Argumedo. "Frequent Behavioral Delay Tendencies by Adults." *Journal of Cross-Cultural Psychology*, 38 (2007): 458–464. DOI: 10.1177/0022022107302314.

Feynman, Richard P. *The Pleasure of Finding Things Out: The Best Short Works of Richard P. Feynman* (Long Island City, NY: Helix Books, 1999).

Fissler, Patrick, Olivia Caroline Küster, Daria Laptinskaya, Laura Sophia Loy, Christine A. F. von Arnim, and Iris-Tatjana Kolassa. "Jigsaw Puzzling Taps Multiple Cognitive Abilities and Is a Potential Protective Factor for Cognitive Aging." *Frontiers in Aging Neuroscience* 10 (October 1, 2018): 299. DOI: 10.3389/fnagi.2018.00299, PMID: 30327598, PMCID: PMC6174231.

Fournier, Denise, PhD "The Only Way to Eat an Elephant." *Psychology Today* (April 18, 2018). https://www.psychologytoday.com/us/blog/mindfully-present-fully-alive/201804/the-only-way-eat-elephant#:~:text=Desmond%20Tutu%20once%20wisely%20said,a%20little%20at%20a%20time.

Frankland, Paul W., Sheena A. Josselyn, and Stefan Köhler. "The Neurobiological Foundation of Memory Retrieval." *Nature Neuroscience* 22, no. 10 (October 2019): 1576–1585. PMCID: PMC6903648, NIHMSID: NIHMS1061667, PMID: 31551594.

Franklin, Benjamin. *Poor Richard's Almanac* (Mount Vernon, New York: Peter Pauper Press, 1980).

Frautschy, S. A., W. Hu, P. Kim, S. A. Miller, T. Chu, M. E. Harris-White, and G. M. Cole. "Phenolic Anti-Inflammatory Antioxidant Reversal of A ß-Induced Cognitive Deficits and Neuropathology." *Neurobiology of Aging* 22, no. 6 (2001): 993–1005, https://doi.org/10.1016/S0197-4580(01)00300-1.

Gangwisch, James E., Lauren Hale, Lorena Garcia, Dolores Malaspina, Mark G. Opler, Martha E. Payne, Rebecca C. Rossom, Dorothy Lane. "High Glycemic Index Diet as a Risk Factor for Depression: Analyses from the Women's Health Initiative." *American Journal of Clinical Nutrition* 102, no. 2 (August 2015): 454–463. https://doi.org/10.3945/ajcn.114.103846, PMID: 26109579, PMCID: PMC4515860.

Gärdenfors, Peter. *Conceptual Spaces: The Geometry of Thought* (Cambridge, MA: MIT Press/Bradford Books, 2004).

Gershoff, Elizabeth T. "Spanking and Child Development: We Know Enough Now to Stop Hitting Our Children." *Child Development Perspectives* 7, no. 3 (2013 September 1, 2013): 133–137. https://doi.org/10.1111/cdep

.12038, PMCID: PMC3768154, NIHMSID: NIHMS488975, PMID: 24039629.

Gesme, Dean, and Marian Wiseman. "How to Implement Change in Practice." *Journal Oncology Practice* 6, no. 5 (September 2010): 257–259. DOI: 10.1200/JOP.000089, PMCID: PMC2936472, PMID: 21197191.

Rabinovici, Gil D., MD; Melanie L. Stephens, PhD; and Katherine L. Possin, PhD; "Executive Dysfunction." *Continuum, Behavioral Neurology and Neuropsychiatry* 21, no. 3 (June 2015): 646–659. DOI: 1212/01. CON.0000466658.05156.54, PMCID: PMC4455841, PMID: 26039846.

Ginsburg, Ruth Bader. *Dissent on Gonzales v. Carhart*, 05–380 F.3d 791, 05–1382 435 F. 3d 1163, reversed (Supreme Court of The United States).

Goldberg, Stanley A. *Clinical Intervention: A Philosophy and Methodology for Clinical Practice* (New York: Macmillan, 1993).

———. *Clinical Skills for Speech-Language Pathologists* (San Diego: Singular Publishing, 1997).

———. *Loving, Supporting, and Caring for the Cancer Patient* (Lanham, MD: Rowman & Littlefield, 2016).

———. *Ready to Learn* (New York: Oxford University Press, 2005).

Gómez-Pinilla, Fernando. "Brain Foods: The Effects of Nutrients on Brain Function." *Nature Reviews Neuroscience* 9, no. 7 (July 2008): 568–578. https://doi.org/10.1038/nrn2421, PMID: 18568016, PMCID: PMC2805706.

Goodwin, Bryan, and Kirsten B. Miller. "Creativity Requires a Mix of Skills." *Research Says* 70, no. 5 (February 1, 2013): 80–82.

Gorges, Eric. *A Craftsman's Legacy with Eric Gorges* (PBS). www.craftmanslegacy.com.

Green C. S. and D. Bavelier. "Exercising Your Brain: A Review of Human Brain Plasticity and Training-Induced Learning," *Psychology in Aging* 23, no. 4 (December 2008): 692–701. DOI: 10.1037/a0014345, PMID: 19140641, PMCID: PMC2896818.

Greenwood, Carol E., and Gordon Winocur. "High-Fat Diets, Insulin Resistance and Declining Cognitive Function." *Neurobiology of Aging* 26, no. 1 (2005): 42–45. https://doi.org/10.1016/j.neurobiolaging.2005.08.017, PMID: 16257476.

Grindlay, Benjamin. "Missing the Point: The Effect of Punctuation on Reading Performance." A dissertation submitted in the Department of Psychology, The University of Adelaide (July 2002).

Gudmundsdottir, Helga Rut. "Advances in Music-Reading Research." *Music Education Research* 12, no. 4 (December 2010): 331–338.

Gupta, Sanjay. *Keep Sharp: Build a Better Brain at Any Age* (New York: Simon & Shuster, 2021).

Halperin, Demian. "Environmental Noise and Sleep Disturbances: A Threat to Health?" *Sleep Science* 7, no 4 (2014): 209–212. DOI: 10.1016/j.slsci.2014.11.003, PMID: 26483931, PMCID: PMC4608916.

Handy, Todd C., Michael B. Miller, Bjoern Schott, Neha M. Shroff, Petr Janata, John D. Van Horn, Souheil Inati, Scott T. Grafton, and Michael S. Gazzangia. "Visual Imagery and Memory: Do Retrieval Strategies Affect What the Mind's Eye Sees?" *European Journal of Cognitive Psychology* 16, no. 5 (2004): 631–652.

Heit, Evan. "Brain Imaging, Forward Inference, and Theories of Reasoning." *Frontiers in Human Neuroscience* 8 (January 09, 2015). https://doi.org/10.3389/fnhum.2014.01056.

Helfer, Karen S., Gabrielle R. Merchant, and Peter A. Wasiuk. "Age-Related Changes in Objective and Subjective Speech Perception in Complex Listening Environments." *Journal of Speech, Language, and Hearing Research* 60, no. 10 (October 2017): 3009–3018. https://doi.org/10.1044/2017_JSLHR-H-17-0030, PMCID: PMC5945070, PMID: 29049601.

Höchli, Bettina. Adrian Brügger, and Claude Messner. "How Focusing on Superordinate Goals Motivates Broad, Long-Term Goal Pursuit: A Theoretical Perspective." *Frontiers in Psychology* 9 (2018): 1879. https://doi.org/10.3389/fpsyg.2018.01879, PMCID: PMC6176065, PMID: 30333781.

Hockey, G. R. J. "Compensatory Control in the Regulation of Human Performance Under Stress and High Workload: A Cognitive-Energetical Framework." *Biological Psychology* 45 (1997): 73–93.

Holland, Kimberly. "Life Expectancy and Long-Term Outlook for Alzheimer's Disease." *Healthline* (September 29, 2018). https://www.healthline.com/health/alzheimers-disease/life-expectancy.

Hoque, Enamul, MD. "Memorization: A Proven Method of Learning." *The Journal of Applied Research* 22, no. 3 (2018):142–150.

Hou, Jinghui, Yijie Wu, and Erin Harrell. "Reading on Paper and Screen Among Senior Adults: Cognitive Map and Technophobia." *Frontiers in Psychology* 8 (December 19, 2017): 2,225. DOI: 10.3389/fpsyg.2017.02225, PMCID: PMC5742182, PMID: 29312073.

Hovhannisyan, Mariam, Alex Clarke, Benjamin R. Geib, Rosalie Cicchinelli, Zachary Monge, Tory Worth, Amanda Szymanski, Roberto Cabeza, Simon W. Davis. "The Visual and Semantic Features That Predict Object Memory: Concept Property Norms for 1,000 Object Images." *Memory & Cognition* 49, no. 4 (May 2021): 712–731. DOI: 10.3758/s13421-020-01130-5, PMID: 33469881, PMCID: PMC8081674.

"How Creativity Works in the Brain: Insights from a Santa Fe Institute Working Group." Cosponsored by the National Endowment for the Arts, July 2015. https://www.arts.gov/sites/default/files/how-creativity-works-in-the-brain-report.pdf

Hudspeth, A. J., and Masakazu Konishi. "Auditory Neuroscience: Development, Transduction, and Integration." *PNAS* 97, no. 22 (October 24, 2000): 11690–11691. https://doi.org/10.1073/pnas.97.22.11690.

Huffington, Adrianna. *The Sleep Revolution* (New York: Harmony, 2016).

Husserl, Edmund. *Ideas: General Introduction to Pure Phenomenology* (Mansfield Center, CT: Martino Fine Books, 2017).

Hwang, Fuu-Jiun, Richard H. Roth, Yu-Wei Wu, Yue Sun, Destany K. Kwon, Yu Liu, Jun B. Ding. "Motor Learning Selectively Strengthens Cortical and Striatal Synapses of Motor Engram Neurons." *Neuron Report* 110, no. 17 (July 08, 2022). DOI: https://doi.org/10.1016/j.neuron.2022.06.006.

Institute of Medicine (US) Committee on Military Nutrition Research. *Caffeine for the Sustainment of Mental Task Performance: Formulations for Military Operations.* (Washington, DC: National Academies Press, 2001). https://www.ncbi.nlm.nih.gov/books/NBK223808

Jabeen, Shaista, and Vatsala Thirumalai. "The Interplay Between Electrical and Chemical Synaptogenesis." *Journal of Neurophysiology* 120, no. 4 (October 2018): 1914–1922. DOI: 10.1152/jn.00398.2018, PMCID: PMC6230774, PMID: 30067121.

Jabr, Ferris. "Why Your Brain Needs More Downtime." *Scientific American* (October 15, 2013).

Jafari, Mohammad Javad, Reza Khosrowabadi, Soheila Khodakarim, and Farough Mohammadian. "The Effect of Noise Exposure on Cognitive Performance and Brain Activity Patterns." *Open Access Macedonian Journal of Medical Sciences* 7, no. 17 (September 2019): 2924–2931. DOI: 10.3889/oamjms.2019.742, PMCID: PMC6901841, PMID: 31844459.

Jiyu-Kennett, Roshi. *Zen is Eternal Life*, 4th ed. (Shasta California: Shasta Abbey, 2000).

Johannes, Niklas, Matti Vuorre, and Andrew K. Przybylski. "Video Game Play is Positively Correlated with Well-Being." *Royal Society of Open Science* 17, no. 2 (February 2021). https://doi.org/10.1098/rsos.202049.

Johns Hopkins Hospital. "Exercising for Better Sleep." (November 18, 2022). https://www.hopkinsmedicine.org/health/wellness-and-prevention/exercising-for-better-sleep.

Jonas, Eric and Konrad Paul Kording. "Could a Neuroscientist Understand a Microprocessor?" *PLOS Computational Biology* 13, no. 1. DOI: 10.1371/journal.pcbi.1005268.

Jones, Doug. *Bending Toward Justice: The Birmingham Church Bombing that Changed the Course of Civil Rights* (All Points Books, 2019).

Jonides, John, Richard L. Lewis, Derek Evan Nee, Cindy A. Lustig, Marc G. Berman, Katherine Sledge Moore. "The Mind and Brain of Short-Term Memory." *Annual Review Psychology* 59 (2008):193–224. DOI: 10.1146/annurev.psych.59.103006.093615.

Joseph, James A., Barbara Shukitt-Hale, and Francis C. Lau. "Fruit Polyphenols and Their Effects on Neuronal Signaling and Behavior in Senescence." *Annals of the New York Academy of Sciences* 1100 (2007): 470–485. https://doi.org/10.1196/annals.1395.052.

Kabat-Zinn, Jon. *Mindfulness for Beginners: Reclaiming the Present Moment and Your Life.*" (Boulder, CO: Sounds True, 2016).

Kaku, Michio. *The Future of the Mind: The Scientific Quest to Understand, Enhance, and Empower the Mind* (New York: Doubleday, 2014).

Keller, Kevin Lane. "Consumer Research Insights on Brands and Branding: A JCR Curation." *Journal of Consumer Research* 46, no. 5 (2020): 995–1001. https://doi.org/10.1093/jcr/ucz058.

Kenett, Yoed N., John D. Medaglia, Roger E. Beaty, Qunlin Chen, Richard F. Netzel, Sharon L. Thompson-Schill, Jiang Qiu. "Driving the Brain Towards Creativity and Intelligence: A Network Control Theory Analysis." *Neuropsychologia* 118, part A (2018): 79–90. DOI: 10.1016/j.neuropsychologia.2018.01.001, PMID: 29307585, PMCID: PMC6034981.

Keng, Shian-Ling, Moria J. Smoski, and Clive J. Robins. "Effects of Mindfulness on Psychological Health: A Review of Empirical Studies." *Clinical Psychology Review* 31, no. 6 (2011): 1041–1056. https://doi.org/10.1016/j.cpr.2011.04.006, PMCID: PMC3679190, NIHMSID: NIHMS463108 PMID: 21802619.

Kersting, Kristian. "Machine Learning and Artificial Intelligence: Two Fellow Travelers on the Quest for Intelligent Behavior in Machines." *Frontiers in Big Data* 1 (November 19, 2018). https://doi.org/10.3389/fdata.2018.00006.

Khambadkone, Seva G., Zachary A. Cordner, Faith Dickerson, Emily G. Severance, Emese Prandovszky, Mikhail Pletnikov, Jianchun Ciao, Ye Li, Gretha J. Boersma, C. Conover Talbot Jr., Wayne W. Campbell, Christian S. Wright, C. Evan Siple, Timothy H. Moran, Kellie L. Tamashiro, and Robert H. Yolken. "Nitrated Meat Products are Associated with Mania in Humans and Altered Behavior and Brain Gene Expression in Rats." *Molecular Psychiatry* 25, no. 3 (March 2020): 560–571. https://doi.org/10.1038/s41380-018-0105-6, PMID: 30022042, PMCID: PMC7077736.

Kim, Bong Jik and Seung-Ha Oh. "Age-Related Changes in Cognition and Speech Perception." *Journal of Audiology & Otology* 17, no. 2 (September 2013): 54–58. https://doi.org/10.7874/kja.2013.17.2.54, PMCID: PMC3936542, PMID: 24653907.

Kim, Hyun-Jun, Hyun-Kyung Park, Dae-Woon Lim, Mi-Hyun Choi, Hyun-Joo Kim, In-Hwa Lee, Hyung-Sik Kim, Jin-Seung Choi, Gye-Rae Tack, Soon-Cheol Chung. "Effects of Oxygen Concentration and Flow Rate on Cognitive Ability and Physiological Responses in the Elderly." *Neural Regeneration Research* 8, no. 3 (January 25, 2013): 264–269. DOI: 10.3969/j.issn.1673-5374.2013.03.009, PMID: 25206597, PMCID: PMC4107523.

Kinsey, Amber W. and Michael J. Ormsbee. "The Health Impact of Nighttime Eating: Old and New Perspectives." *Nutrients* 7, no. 4 (2015): 2648–2662.

DOI: https://doi.org/10.3390/nu7042648, PMID: 25859885, PMCID: PMC4425165.

Klatte, Maria, Kirstin Bergström, and Thomas Lachmann. "Does Noise Affect Learning? A Short Review on Noise Effects on Cognitive Performance in Children." *Frontiers in Psychology* 4 (August 2013): 578. DOI: 10.3389/fpsyg.2013.00578, PMCID: PMC3757288, PMID: 24009598.

Kondo, Marie. *The Life-Changing Magic of Tidying Up: The Japanese Art of Decluttering and Organizing* (Emeryville, CA: Ten Speed Press, 2014).

Krishnamurti, J. *Think on These Things* (New York, NY: Harper and Row, 1964).

Kryscio, Richard J., Erin L. Abner, Gregory E. Cooper, David W. Fardo, Gregory A. Jicha, Peter T. Nelson, Charles D. Smith, Linda J. Van Eldik, Lijie Wan, Frederick A. Schmitt. "Self-Reported Memory Complaints: Implications From a Longitudinal Cohort with Autopsies." *Neurology* 83, no. 15 (September 2014): 1359–1365. https://doi.org/10.1212/WNL .0000000000000856, PMID: 25253756, PMCID: PMC4189103.

Kühn, S., A. Romanowski, C. Schilling, R. Lorenz, C. Mörsen, N. Seiferth, T. Banaschewski, A Barbot, G J Barker, C Büchel, P J Conrod, J W Dalley, H Flor, H Garavan, B. Ittermann, K. Mann, J.-L. Martinot, T. Paus, M. Rietschel, M. N. Smolka, A. Ströhle, B. Walaszek, G. Schumann, A. Heinz, and J. Gallinat. "The Neural Basis of Video Gaming." *Translational Psychiatry* 1, no. 53 (November 15, 2011). https://doi.org/10.1038/tp.2011.53.

Kume, June. "Meditation and Mindfulness Peer-Reviewed Literature: Review." *Journal of Yoga and Physiotherapy* 5, no. 4 (July 17, 2018). DOI:10.19080/ JYP.2018.05.555669.

Lacy, Joyce W., and Craig E. L. Stark. "The Neuroscience of Memory: Implications for the Courtroom." *Nature Reviews Neuroscience* 14, no. 9 (2013): 649–658. DOI: 10.1038/nrn3563, PMCID: PMC4183265, PMID: 23942467.

Lally, Phillippa, Cornelia H. M. van Jaarsveld, Henry W. W. Potts, and Jan Wardle. "How Are Habits Formed: Modelling Habit Formation in the Real World." *European Journal of Social Psychology* 40, no. 6 (July 16, 2009): 998–1009. https://doi.org/10.1002/ejsp.674.

Lateef, Fatimah. "Simulation-Based Learning: Just Like the Real Thing." *Journal of Emergencies, Trauma, and Shock* 3, no. 4 (2010): 348–352. DOI: 10.4103/0974-2700.70743, PMCID: PMC2966567, PMID: 21063557.

Lehmann, Janina A. M., and Tina Seufert. "The Influence of Background Music on Learning in the Light of Different Theoretical Perspectives and the Role of Working Memory Capacity." *Frontiers in Psychology* 8 (October 31, 2017). https://doi.org/10.3389/fpsyg.2017.01902, PMCID: PMC5671572, PMID: 29163283.

Leonard, Jay. "Why Do Customers Hate Your Offshore Call Center So Much?" *Business 2 Community* (January 2023). https://www.business2community

.com/customer-experience/customers-hate-offshore-call-center-much
-0855971.

Letenneur, L., C. Proust-Lima, A. Le Gouge, J.F. Dartigues, and P. Barberg-er-Gateau. "Flavonoid Intake and Cognitive Decline Over a 10-Year Period." *American Journal of Epidemiology* 165, no. 12 (2007): 1364–1371. https://doi.org/10.1093/aje/kwm036.

Levi, Susannah V., Stephen J. Winters, David B. Pisoni. "Effects of Cross-Language Voice Training on Speech Perception: Whose Familiar Voices Are More Intelligible?" *Journal of the Acoustical Society of America* 13, no. 6 (December 2011): 4053–4062. DOI: 10.1121/1.3651816, PMCID: PMC3253604, PMID: 22225059.

Lilly, Kelsey. "Chaining Techniques: A Systematic Literature Review and Best Practice Recommendations." *Culminating Projects in Community Psychology, Counseling and Family Therapy* 74 (2020). https://repository.stcloudstate.edu/cpcf_etds/74.

Lisman, John. "The Challenge of Understanding the Brain: Where We Stand in 2015." *Neuron* 86, no. 4 (May 2015): 864–882. DOI: 10.1016/j.neuron.2015.03.032, PMID: 25996132, PMCID: PMC4441769.

Lohmann, Robert. "Effects of Simulation-Based Learning and One Way to Analyze Them." *Journal of Political Science Education* 16, no. 4 (2020): 479–495. https://doi.org/10.1080/15512169.2019.1599291.

Lonky, Martin L. "Human Consciousness: A Systems Approach to the Mind/Brain Interaction." *Journal of Mind & Behavior* 24, no. 1 (Winter 2003): 91–118.

Lourenco, Frederico, and B. J. Casey. "Adjusting Behavior to Changing Environmental Demands with Development." *Neuroscience and Biobehavorial Reviews* 37, 9, part B (2013): 2233–42. DOI: 10.1016/j.neubiorev.2013.03.003, PMCID: PMC3751996, PMID: 23518271, NIHMSID: NIHMS459426.

Lucassen, Paul J., Jens Pruessner, Nuno Sousa, Osborne F. X. Almeida, Anne Marie Van Dam, Grazyna Rajkowska, Dick F. Swaab, and Boldizsár Czéh. "Neuropathology of Stress." *Acta Neuropathologica* 127, no. 1 (2014): 109–135. DOI: 10.1007/s00401-013-1223-5, PMCID: PMC3889685, PMID: 24318124.

Lum, Jarrad A. G., and Gina Conti-Ramsden. "Long-Term Memory: A Review and Meta-Analysis of Studies of Declarative and Procedural Memory in Specific Language Impairment." *Topics in Language Disorders* 33, no. 4 (December 1, 2013): 282–297. https://doi.org/10.1097/01.tld.0000437939.01237.6a, PMCID: PMC3986888, EMSID: EMS57240, PMID: 24748707.

MacLeod, Sydney, Michael G. Reynolds, and Hugo Lehmann. "The Mitigating Effect of Repeated Memory Reactivations on Forgetting." *NPJ Science of*

Learning 3, article 9 (April 2018). https://doi.org/10.1038/s41539-018 -0025-x.

Maguire, Eleanor A., David G. Gadian, Ingrid S. Johnsrude, Catriona D. Good, John Ashburner, Richard S. J. Frackowiak, and Christopher D. Frith. "Navigation-Related Structural Change in the Hippocampi of Taxi Drivers." *PNAS* 97, no. 8 (2000): 4398–4403. https://doi.org/10.1073/pnas .070039597.

Mah, Yee-Haur, Masud Husain, Geraint Rees, Parashkev Nachev. "Human Brain Lesion-Deficit Inference Remapped." *Brain* 137, no. 9 (September 2014): 2522–2531. https://doi.org/10.1093/brain/awu164.

Mandolesi, Laura, Arianna Polverino, Simone Montuori, Francesca Foti, Giampaolo Ferraioli, Pierpaolo Sorrentino, and Giuseppe Sorrentino. "Effects of Physical Exercise on Cognitive Functioning and Wellbeing: Biological and Psychological Benefits." *Frontiers in Psychology* 9 (April 27, 2018). https://doi.org/10.3389/fpsyg.2018.00509, PMCID: PMC593499, PMID: 29755380.

Manohar, Sanjay G., Yoni Pertzov, and Masud Husain. "Short-Term Memory for Spatial, Sequential and Duration Information." *Current Opinion Behavioral Sciences* 17 (October 2017): 20–26. DOI: 10.1016/j. cobeha.2017.05.023, PMCID: PMC5678495, PMID: 29167809.

Maraboli, Steve. *Life, the Truth, and Being Free* (Port Washington, NY: Better Today Publishing, November 10, 2009).

Marrufo-Pérez, Miriam I., Almudena Eustaquio-Martín, and Enrique A. Lopez-Poveda. "Adaptation to Noise in Human Speech Recognition Unrelated to the Medial Olivocochlear Reflex." *Journal of Neuroscience* 38, no. 17 (April 25, 2018): 4138–4145. https://doi.org/10.1523/jneurosci .0024-18.2018.

Marrufo-Pérez, Miriam I., Dora del Pilar Sturla-Carreto, Almudena Eustaquio-Martín and Enrique A. Lopez-Poveda. "Adaptation to Noise in Human Speech Recognition Depends on Noise-Level Statistics and Fast Dynamic-Range Compression." *Journal of Neuroscience* 40, no. 34 (August 19, 2020): 6613–6623. https://doi.org/10.1523/JNEUROSCI .0469-20.2020.

Martins, Isabel Pavão, Rosário Vieira, Clara Loureiro, and M. Emilia Santos. "Speech Rate and Fluency in Children and Adolescents." *Child Neuropsychology* 13, no. 4 (June 12, 2007): 319–332. https://doi.org/10.1080 /09297040600837370.

Mattson, Mark P. "Superior Pattern Processing Is the Essence of the Evolved Human Brain." *Frontiers in Neuroscience* 8 (August 22, 2014): 265. DOI: 10.3389/fnins.2014.00265, PMID: 25202234, PMCID: PMC4141622.

McCann, Joyce C. and Bruce N. Ames. "Is Docosahexaenoic Acid, an N-3 Long-Chain Polyunsaturated Fatty Acid, Required for Development of Normal Brain Function? An Overview of Evidence from Cognitive and

Behavioral Tests in Humans and Animals." *American Journal of Clinical Nutrition* 82, no. 2 (2005): 281–295. https://doi.org/10.1093/ajcn.82.2 .281, PMID: 16087970.

Mcleod, Saul. "What is Cognitive Dissonance? Definition and Examples," *Simply Psychology* (March 6, 2023).

Metcalfe, Janet. "Learning from Errors," *Annual Review of Psychology* 68, no. 1 (2017): 465–489

Medic, Goran, Micheline Wille, Michiel Eh Hemels. "Short- and Long-Term Health Consequences of Sleep Disruption." *Nature and Science of Sleep* 19, no. 9 (2017): 151–161. https://doi.org/10.2147/NSS.S134864, PMID: 28579842, PMCID: PMC5449130.

Melis, René J. F., Miriam L. Haaksma, Graciela Muniz-Terrera. "Understanding and Predicting the Longitudinal Course of Dementia." *Current Opinion in Psychiatry* 32, no. 2 (2019): 123–129. https://doi.org/10.1097/YCO .0000000000000482, PMCID: PMC6380437, PMID: 30557268.

Middleton, Sophie, Alexandra Charnock, Sarah Forster, and John Blakey. "Factors Affecting Individual Task Prioritisation in a Workplace Setting." *Future Healthcare Journal* 5, no. 2 (June 2018): 138–142. https://doi.org/10 .7861/futurehosp.5-2-138, PMID: 31098549, PMCID: PMC6502562.

Mikneviciute, Greta, Nicola Ballhausen, Ulrike Rimmele, Matthias Kliegel. "Does Older Adults' Cognition Particularly Suffer from Stress? A Systematic Review of Acute Stress Effects on Cognition in Older Age." *Neuroscience & Biobehavioral Reviews* 132 (January 2022): 583–602.

Mills, Kyle. "The 10 Secrets of Success by Bob Bowman." *American Swimming Coaches Association* (January 2017).

Moeser, Shannon Dawn. "Memory for Meaning and Wording in Concrete and Abstract Sentences." *Journal of Verbal Learning and Verbal Behavior* 13, no. 6 (December 1974): 682–697.

Mograbi, Daniel C., Robin G. Morris. "Anosognosia." *Cortex: A Journal Devoted to the Study of the Nervous System and Behavior* 103 (June 2018): 385–386. https://doi.org/10.1016/j.cortex.2018.04.001, PMID: 29731103.

Mohr, Peter N. C., and Irene E. Nagel. "Variability in Brain Activity as an Individual Difference Measure in Neuroscience?" *Journal of Neuroscience* 30, no. 23 (June 9, 2010): 7755–7757. https://doi.org/10.1523/JNEUROSCI .1560-10.2010.

Moisala, M., V. Salmela, L. Hietajärvi, S. Carlson, V. Vuontela, K. Lonka, K. Hakkarainen, K. Salmela-Aro, K. Alho. "Gaming is Related to Enhanced Working Memory Performance and Task-Related Cortical Activity." *Brain Research* 1655 (January 15, 2017): 204–215. DOI: 10.1016/j. brainres.2016.10.027.

Monty Python. "Mr. Creosote, full version." YouTube. https://www.youtube.com /watch?v=GxRnenQYG7I.

Murayama, Kou, Adam B. Blake, Tyson Kerr, Alan D. Castel. "When Enough Is Not Enough: Information Overload and Metacognitive Decisions to Stop Studying Information." *Journal of Experimental Psychology, Learning, Memory, and Cognition* 42, no. 6 (June 2016): 914–924. DOI: 10.1037/xlm0000213, PMCID: PMC4877291, NIHMSID: NIHMS732615, PMID: 26595067.

Murman, Daniel L. "The Impact of Age on Cognition." *Seminars in Hearing* 36, no. 3 (August 2015): 111–121. DOI: 10.1055/s-0035-1555115, PMCID: PMC4906299, PMID: 27516712.

Nassiff, Peter J. and E. R. Boyko. "Teaching the Method of Successive Approximations." *Journal of Chemical Education* 55, no. 6 (June 1, 1978): 376. https://doi.org/10.1021/ed055p376.

National Institutes of Health. "Alzheimer's Disease" (2018). https://www.nih.gov/research-training/accelerating-medicines-partnership-amp/alzheimers-disease.

Newkirk, Thomas. "The Case for Slow Reading." *Educational Leadership* 67, no 6 (March 2010): 6–11.

Nobre, Anna Christina and Freek van Ede. "Under the Mind's Hood: What We Have Learned by Watching the Brain at Work." *Journal of Neuroscience* 40, no. 1 (January 2020), 89–100. https://doi.org/10.1523/jneurosci.0742-19.2019.

Ohsugi, Hironori, Shohei Ohgi, Kenta Shigemori, and Eric B. Schneider. "Differences in Dual-Task Performance and Prefrontal Cortex Activation Between Younger and Older Adults." *BMC Neuroscience* 14, no. 10 (January 18, 2013). https://doi.org/10.1186/1471-2202-14-10.

Okamoto-Mizuno, Kazue and Koh Mizuno. "Effects of Thermal Environment on Sleep and Circadian Rhythm." *Journal of Physiological Anthropology* 31, no. 14 (2012). https://doi.org/10.1186/1880-6805-31-14, PMID: 22738673, PMCID: PMC3427038.

Oppezzo, Marily, and Daniel L. Schwartz. "Give Your Ideas Some Legs: The Positive Effect of Walking on Creative Thinking." *Journal of Experimental Psychology: Learning, Memory, and Cognition* 40, no. 4 (2014): 1142–1152.

Pacheco, Danielle. "Alcohol and Sleep." *Sleep Foundation*, September 19, 2022.

———. "The Best Temperature for Sleep." The Sleep Foundation (September 29, 2022). https://www.sleepfoundation.org/bedroom-environment/best-temperature-for-sleep#:~:text=A%20National%20Sleep%20Foundation%20poll,Fahrenheit%20(18.3%20degrees%20Celsius).

Pagel, J. F., Bennett L. Parnes. "Medications for the Treatment of Sleep Disorders: An Overview." *Primary Care Companion to the Journal of Clinical Psychiatry* 3, no. 3 (2001): 118–125. DOI: 10.4088/pcc.v03n0303, PMID: 15014609, PMCID: PMC181172.

Park, Soon-Yeob, Mi-Kyeong Oh, Bum-Soon Lee, Haa-Gyoung Kim, Won-Joon Lee, Ji-Ho Lee, Jun-Tae Lim, Jin-Young Kim. "The Effects of Alcohol on

Quality of Sleep." *Korean Journal of Family Medicine* 36, no. 6 (2015): 294–9. https://doi.org/10.4082/kjfm.2015.36.6.294, PMID: 26634095, PMCID: PMC4666864.

Parekh, Diva. "Learning to Listen to My Mind and My Body." *Johns Hopkins News-Letter* (January 30, 2020).

Pearson, Keith E., Virginia G. Wadley, Leslie A. McClure, James M. Shikany, Fred W. Unverzagt, and Suzanne E. Judd. "Dietary Patterns Are Associated with Cognitive Function in the Reasons for Geographic and Racial Differences in Stroke (REGARDS) Cohort." *Journal of Nutritional Science* 5, no. 38 (2016). https://doi.org/10.1017/jns.2016.27, PMID: 27752305, PMCID: PMC5048188.

Pendrya, Louise F. and Jessica Salvatore. "Individual and Social Benefits of Online Discussion Forums." *Computers in Human Behavior* 50 (September 2015): 211–220. https://doi.org/10.1016/j.chb.2015.03.067.

Penny, Rick. "Three Components of a Quick Release: How Stephen Curry & Melissa Dixon Use Them to Their Advantage." *Breakthrough Basketball* 13 (Oct 2022).

Perkins, Anthony J., Hugh C. Hendrie, Christopher M. Callahan, Sujuan Gao, Frederick W. Unverzagt, Yong Xu, Kathleen S. Hall, Siu L. Hui. "Association of Antioxidants with Memory in a Multiethnic Elderly Sample Using the Third National Health and Nutrition Examination Survey." *American Journal of Epidemiology* 150, no. 1, (1999): 37–44. https://doi.org/10.1093/oxfordjournals.aje.a009915.

Perlovsky, Leonid. "A Challenge to Human Evolution-Cognitive Dissonance," *Frontiers in Psychology* 4 (April 10, 2013):179. DOI: 10.3389/fpsyg.2013.00179, PMID: 23596433, PMCID: PMC3622034.

Pietilä, Julia. Elina Helander, Ilkka Korhonen, Tero Myllymäki, Harri Lindholm. "Acute Effect of Alcohol Intake on Cardiovascular Autonomic Regulation During the First Hours of Sleep in a Large Real-World Sample of Finnish Employees: Observational Study." *JMIR Mental Health* 5, no. 1 (2018). https://doi.org/10.2196/mental.9519, PMID: 29549064, PMCID: PMC5878366.

Pisoni, David B. "Speech Perception: Some New Directions in Research and Theory." *Journal of the Acoustical Society of America* 78, no. 1, pt. 2 (July 1985): 381–388. https://doi.org/10.1121/1.392451, PMCID: PMC3517998, NIHMSID: NIHMS418763, PMID: 4031245.

Pitt, Mark A. "How Are Pronunciation Variants of Spoken Words Recognized? A Test of Generalization to Newly Learned Words." *Journal of Memory and Language* 61, no. 1 (July 2009): 19–36. DOI: 10.1016/j.jml.2009.02.005, PMID: 20161243, PMCID: PMC2706522.

Pninit, Russo-Netzer. "Prioritizing Meaning as a Pathway to Meaning in Life and Well-Being." *Journal of Happiness Studies* 20, no. 2 (August 2019). DOI:10.1007/s10902-018-0031-y.

Popkin, Barry M., Kristen E. D'Anci, Irwin H. Rosenberg. "Water, Hydration, and Health." *Nutrition Reviews* 68, no. 8 (August 2010): 439–458. https://doi.org/10.1111/j.1753-4887.2010.00304.x, PMID: 20646222, PMCID: PMC2908954.

"Prostate Cancer: The Gleason Score Explained." Fox Chase Cancer Center, Temple University, July 26, 2018. https://www.foxchase.org/blog/prostate-cancer-gleason-score-explained.

Pruitt, Sarah. "Why Does the Leaning Tower of Pisa Lean?" https://www.history.com/news/why-does-the-leaning-tower-of-pisa-lean.

Przybelski, Robert J. and Neil C. Binkley. "Is Vitamin D Important for Preserving Cognition? A Positive Correlation of Serum 25-Hydroxyvitamin D Concentration with Cognitive Function." *Archives of Biochemistry and Biophysics* 460, no. 2 (2007): 202–205. https://doi.org/10.1016/j.abb.2006.12.018.

Pusch, Roland, Julian Packheiser, Amir Hossein Azizi, Celil Semih Sevincik, Jonas Rose, Sen Cheng, Maik C. Stüttgen, Onur Güntürkün. "Working Memory Performance is Tied to Stimulus Complexity." *bioRxiv* (2021). https://doi.org/10.1101/2021.09.10.459776.

Puthusseryppady, Vaisakh, Luke Emrich-Mills, Ellen Lowry, Martyn Patel, and Michael Hornberger. "Spatial Disorientation in Alzheimer's Disease: The Missing Path from Virtual Reality to Real World." *Frontiers in Aging Neuroscience* 12 (October 27, 2020): 550514. https://doi.org/10.3389/fnagi.2020.550514, PMCID: PMC7652847, PMID: 33192453.

Quinn, J. L. and Will Cresswell. "Predator Hunting Behaviour and Prey Vulnerability." *Journal of Animal Ecology* 73, no. 1 (2004): 143–154. https://www.jstor.org/stable/3505324.

Rasch, Björn and Jan Born. "About Sleep's Role in Memory." *Physiological Reviews* 93, no. 2 (April 2013): 681–766. DOI: 10.1152/physrev.00032.2012, PMCID: PMC3768102, PMID: 23589831.

Reagh, Zachariah M., Jessica A. Noche, Nicholas J. Tustison, Derek Delisle, Elizabeth A. Murray, Michael A. Yassa. "Functional Imbalance of Anterolateral Entorhinal Cortex and Hippocampal Dentate/CA3 Underlies Age-Related Object Pattern Separation Deficits." *Neuron* 97, no. 5 (March 2018): 1187–1198. https://doi.org/10.1016/j.neuron.2018.01.039, PMID: 29518359, PMCID: PMC5937538.

Regopoulos, M. "The Principle of Causation as a Basis of Scientific Method." *Management Science* 12, no. 8, (April 1966), B-287–C-177. https://doi.org/10.1287/mnsc.12.8.C135.

Richards, Regina G. "Making It Stick: Memorable Strategies to Enhance Learning." LD Online (2008). http://www.ldonline.org/article/5602.

Richardson, Michael W. "How Much Energy Does the Brain Use?" *BrainFacts.org*, (February 2, 2019).

Robinson, R. "Cost-Benefit Analysis." *BMJ* 307, no. 6909 (October 1993): 924–926. https://doi.org/10.1136/bmj.307.6909.924, PMCID: PMC1679054, PMID: 8241859.

Rosi, Alessia, Elena Cavallini, Nadia Gamboz, Tomaso Vecchi, Floris Tijmen Van Vugt, and Riccardo Russo. "The Impact of Failures and Successes on Affect and Self-Esteem in Young and Older Adults." *Frontiers in Psychology* 10 (August 6, 2019). https://doi.org/10.3389/fpsyg.2019.01795.

Rubel, Robert C. "The Epistemology of War Gaming." *Naval War College Review* 59, no. 2, article 8 (2006). https://digital-commons.usnwc.edu/nwc-review/vol59/iss2/8.

Ruff, Holly A., and Mary C. Capozzoli. "The Development of Attention and Distractibility in the First 4 Years of Life." *Developmental Psychology* 39 (September 2003): 877–90.

Rumar, Kåre. "The Role of Perceptual and Cognitive Filters in Observed Behavior." *Human Behavior and Traffic Safety*, eds. Leonard Evans and Richard C. Schwing (Boston: Springer, 1985). https://doi.org/10.1007/978-1-4613-2173-6_8.

Sagan, Carl. *Cosmos* (New York: Random House, 1983).

Sala, Giovanni, John P. Foley, and Fernand Gobet. "The Effects of Chess Instruction on Pupils' Cognitive and Academic Skills: State of the Art and Theoretical Challenges." *Frontiers in Psychology* 8 (February 23, 2017). https://doi.org/10.3389/fpsyg.2017.00238, PMID: 28280476; PMCID: PMC5322219.

Sander, Elizabeth J., Arran Caza, and Peter J. Jordan. "Psychological Perceptions Matter: Developing the Reactions to the Physical Work Environment Scale." *Building and Environment* 148, no. 15 (January 2019): 338–347. https://doi.org/10.1016/j.buildenv.2018.11.020.

Schwarz, Allan B. "Medical Mystery: Did Reagan have Alzheimer's While President?" *Philadelphia Inquirer* (August 13, 2016).

Sege, Robert D., MD, and Benjamin S. Siegel, MD. "Effective Discipline to Raise Healthy Children." *Pediatrics* 142, no. 6 (December 2018). https://doi.org/10.1542/peds.2018-3112.

Seger, Carol A., and Earl K. Miller. "Category Learning in the Brain." *Annual Review of Neuroscience* 33 (July 21, 2010): 203–19. DOI: 10.1146/annurev.neuro.051508.135546, PMID: 20572771, PMCID: PMC3709834.

Seli, Paul, Brandon C. W. Ralph, Evan F. Risko, Jonathan W. Schooler, Daniel L. Schacter, Daniel Smilek. "Intentionality and Meta-Awareness of Mind Wandering: Are They One and the Same, or Distinct Dimensions?" *Psychonomic Bulletin & Review* 24, no. 6 (December 2017): 1808–1818. DOI: 10.3758/s13423-017-1249-0, PMID: 28244016, PMCID: PMC5572547.

Servant, Mathieu, Peter Cassey, Geoffrey F. Woodman, Gordon D. Logan. "Neural Bases of Automaticity." *Journal of Experimental Psychology, Learning, Memory, and Cognition* 44, no. 3 (2018): 440–464. DOI: 10.1037/

xlm0000454, PMCID: PMC5862722, NIHMSID: NIHMS894496, PMID: 28933906.

Sexton, Claire E., Andreas B. Storsve, Kristine B. Walhovd, Heidi Johansen-Berg, Anders M. Fjell. "Poor Sleep Quality is Associated with Increased Cortical Atrophy in Community-Dwelling Adults." *Neurology* 83, no. 11 (September 9, 2014): 967–973. https://doi.org/10.1212/WNL .0000000000000774.

Shah, Carolin, Katharina Erhard, Hanns-Joseph Ortheil, Evangelia Kaza, Christof Kessler, and Martin Lotze. "Neural Correlates of Creative Writing: An fMRI Study." *Human Brain Mapping* 34, no. 5 (May 2013): 1088–101. DOI: 10.1002/hbm.21493, PMID: 22162145, PMCID: PMC6869990.

Shakespeare, William. *Macbeth* (Wordsworth Classics, 1992).

Shechter, Ari, Elijah W. Kim, Marie-Pierre St-Onge, Andrew J. Westwood. "Blocking Nocturnal Blue Light for Insomnia: A Randomized Controlled Trial." *Journal of Psychiatric Research* 96 (2018): 196–202. DOI: 10.1016/j. jpsychires.2017.10.015, PMID: 29101797, PMCID: PMC5703049.

Sherman, Jeremy E., PhD. "Psychological Crutches: Ten Myths and Three Tips." *Psychology Today* (April 17, 2014). https://www.psychologytoday .com/us/blog/ambigamy/201404/psychological-crutches-ten-myths-and -three-tips.

Sherwood, Chet C., Francys Subiaul, Tadeusz W. Zawidzki. "A Natural History of the Human Mind: Tracing Evolutionary Changes in Brain and Cognition." *Journal of Anatomy* 212, no. 4 (April 2008): 426–54. DOI: 10.1111/j.1469-7580.2008.00868.x, PMID: 18380864, PMCID: PMC2409100.

Shokri-Kojori, Ehsan, Gene-Jack Wang, Corinde E. Wiers, Sukru B. Demiral, Min Guo, Sung Won Kim, Elsa Lindgren, Veronica Ramirez, Amna Zehra, Clara Freeman, Gregg Miller, Peter Manza, Tansha Srivastava, Susan De Santi, Dardo Tomasi, Helene Benveniste, and Nora D. Volkow. "ß-Amyloid Accumulation in the Human Brain After One Night of Sleep Deprivation." *Proceedings of the National Academy of Sciences* (PNAS) 115, no. 17, (April 9, 2018): 4483–4488. https://doi.org/10.1073/pnas .1721694115, PMID: 29632177.

Skinner, B.F. *Science and Human Behavior* (New York: Free Press, 1965).

Smith, Steven M., and Arthur Glenberg. "Environmental Context and Human Memory." *Memory & Cognition* 6, no. 4 (1978): 342–353.

Sokol, Justin T. "Identity Development Throughout the Lifetime: An Examination of Eriksonian Theory." *Graduate Journal of Counseling Psychology* 1, no. 2, article 14, (2009). http://epublications.marquette.edu/gjcp/vol1/iss2/14.

Sorrell, Jeanne M. "Tidying Up: Good for the Aging Brain." *Journal of Psychosocial Nursing and Mental Health Services* 58, no. 4 (2020): 16–18. DOI: 10.3928/02793695-20200316-02, PMID: 32219461.

Squire, Larry R. "Memory and Brain Systems: 1969–2009." *Journal of Neuroscience* 29, no. 41 (October 14, 2009): 12711–12716. https://doi.org/10.1523/JNEUROSCI.3575-09.2009.

Squire, Larry R., Lisa Genzel, John T. Wixted, Richard G. Morris. "Memory Consolidation." *Cold Spring Harbor Perspectives in Biology* 7, no. 8 (August 3, 2015). DOI: 10.1101/cshperspect.a021766, PMCID: PMC4526749, PMID: 26238360.

Steenbergen, Laura, Roberta Sellaro, Ann-Kathrin Stock, Christian Beste, Lorenza S. Colzato. "Action Video Gaming and Cognitive Control: Playing First Person Shooter Games Is Associated with Improved Action Cascading but Not Inhibition." *PLoS ONE* 10, no. 12 (2015). https://doi.org/10.1371/journal.pone.0144364.

Stephens, Greg J., Lauren J. Silbert, and Uri Hasson. "Speaker-Listener Neural Coupling Underlies Successful Communication." *Proceedings of the National Academy of Sciences of the United States of America* 107, no. 32 (August 10, 2010): 14425–30.

"Stephen Curry Has Hit 42.8 Percent of His Threes in His Career." *Statmuse* 15 (October 2022). https://www.statmuse.com/nba/ask/steph-curry-career-3pt-percentage.

Tajfe, Henri. *Human Groups and Social Categories: Studies in Social Psychology* (Cambrige: Cambridge University Press, 1981).

Tallberg, I. M., and G. Bergendal. "Strategies of Lexical Substitution and Retrieval in Multiple Sclerosis." *Aphasiology*, 23, no. 9 (2009): 1184–1195. DOI: 10.1080/02687030802436884.

Tarawneh, Rawan, and David M. Holtzman. "The Clinical Problem of Symptomatic Alzheimer Disease and Mild Cognitive Impairment." *Cold Spring Harbor Perspectives in Medicine* 2, no. 5 (May 2012). DOI:10.1101/cshperspect.a006148.

Tavakoli, Elahe, and Shiela Kheirzadeh. "The Effect of Font Size on Reading Comprehension Skills: Scanning for Key Words and Reading for General Idea." *Theory and Practice in Language Studies* 1, no. 7 (July 2011): 915–919. DOI: 10.4304/tpls.1.7.915-919.

Teki, Sundeep, Maria Chait, Sukhbinder Kumar, Katharina von Kriegstein and Timothy D. Griffiths. "Brain Bases for Auditory Stimulus-Driven Figure—Ground Segregation." *Journal of Neuroscience* 31, no. 1 (January 5, 2011): 164–171. https://doi.org/10.1523/JNEUROSCI.3788-10.2011.

Tell, Phillip M. "Influence of Vocalization on Short-Term Memory." *Journal of Verbal Learning and Verbal Behavior* 10, no. 2 (1971): 149–156.

Therriault, Joseph, Kok Pin Ng, Tharick A. Pascoal, Sulantha Mathotaarachchi, Min Su Kang, Hanne Struyfs, Monica Shin, Andrea L. Benedet, Ishan C. Walpola, Vasavan Nair, Serge Gauthier, Pedro Rosa-Neto. "Anosognosia Predicts Default Mode Network Hypometabolism and

Clinical Progression to Dementia." *Neurology* 90, no. 11 (2018). https://doi.org/10.1212/WNL.0000000000005120, PMID: 29444971, PMCID: PMC5858945.

Todorov, Ivo, Fabio Del Missier, and Timo Mäntylä. "Age-Related Differences in Multiple Task Monitoring." *PLoS One* 9, no. 9 (September 12, 2014): e107619. DOI: 10.1371/journal.pone.0107619, PMID: 25215609, PMCID: PMC4162647.

Tosini, Gianluca, Ian Ferguson, and Kazuo Tsubota. "Effects of Blue Light on the Circadian System and Eye Physiology." *Molecular Vision* 22 (2016): 61–72, PMID: 26900325, PMCID: PMC4734149.

Trafton, Anne. "Neuroscientists Reveal How the Brain Can Enhance Connections: Newly Identified Mechanism Allows the Brain to Strengthen Links Between Neurons." *MIT News.* https://news.mit.edu/2015/brain-strengthen-connections-between-neurons-1118.

Travica, Nikolaj, Karin Ried, Avni Sali, Andrew Scholey, Irene Hudson, and Andrew Pipingas. "Vitamin C Status and Cognitive Function: A Systematic Review." *Nutrients* 9, no. 9 (August 2017): 960. https://doi.org/10.3390/nu9090960, PMID: 28867798, PMCID: PMC5622720.

Tripathy, Srimant P., and Haluk Öğmen. "Sensory Memory Is Allocated Exclusively to the Current Event-Segment." *Frontiers in Psychology* 9 (September 7, 2018). https://doi.org/10.3389/fpsyg.2018.01435.

Tyson, Neil DeGrasse. "How Does the Brain Work?" *NOVA scienceNOW,* www.pbs.org. September 14, 2011.

———. "NFL Films Present—Keep Running." October 10, 2022.

The Ultimate Popeye Collection (1933–1945) with 138 Original, Remastered, Uncut Cartoons & Theatrical Shorts and Loaded w/ Bonus Content! (Fletcher Studios).

Van Cauter, Eve, Daniel Désir, Christine Decoster, Franchise Féry, and Edmond O. Balasse. "Nocturnal Decrease in Glucose Tolerance During Constant Glucose Infusion." *Journal of Clinical Endocrinology & Metabolism* 69, no. 3 (1989): 604–611. https://doi.org/10.1210/jcem-69-3-604.

Vasic, Verica, Kathrin Barth, and Mirko H. H. Schmidt. "Neurodegeneration and Neuro–Regeneration–Alzheimer's Disease and Stem Cell Therapy." *International Journal of Molecular Sciences* 20, no. 17 (August 31, 2019): 4272. https://doi.org/10.3390/ijms20174272, PMCID: PMC6747457, PMID: 31480448.

Vasilev, Martin R., Julie A. Kirkby, and Bernhard Angele. "Auditory Distraction During Reading: A Bayesian Meta-Analysis of a Continuing Controversy." *Perspectives on Psychological Science: A Journal of the Association for Psychological Science* 13, no. 5 (2018): 567–597. DOI:10.1177/1745691617747398, PMID: 29958067, PMCID: PMC6139986.

Vilaverde, Daniela, Jorge Gonçalves, and Pedro Morgado. "Hoarding Disorder: A Case Report." *Frontiers in Psychiatry* 8 (June 28, 2017): 112. DOI: 10.3389/fpsyt.2017.00112, PMCID: PMC5487393, PMID: 28701963.

Von Moltke, Helmuth, *Moltke on the Art of War: Selected Writings*, Daniel Hughes (ed) (Presidio Press, 1995.)

Wammes, Jeffrey D., Brady R. T. Roberts, and Myra A. Fernandes. "Task Preparation as a Mnemonic: The Benefits of Drawing (and Not Drawing)." *Psychonomic Bulletin & Review* 25, no. 6 (2018): 2365–2372. DOI: 10.3758/s13423-018-1477-y.

Warner, Natasha, Dan Brenner, Benjamin V. Tucker, and Mirjam Ernestus. "Native Listeners' Use of Information in Parsing Ambiguous Casual Speech." *Brain Sciences* 12, no. 7 (July 15, 2022): 930. https: //doi.org/10.3390/brainsci12070930.

Watts, Michelle E., Roger Pocock, and Charles Claudianos. "Brain Energy and Oxygen Metabolism: Emerging Role in Normal Function and Disease." *Frontiers in Molecular Neuroscience* 22 (June 2018). https://doi.org/10.3389/fnmol.2018.00216.

Welch, Jack. *Winning* (New York: Harper Business, 2005).

Wilcox, James A., and Reid Duffy. "Is It a 'Senior Moment' or Early Dementia? Addressing Memory Concerns in Older Patients." *Current Psychiatry* 15, no. 5 (May 2016): 28–30, 32–34, 40.

Wilms, Inge L., Anders Petersen, and Signe Vangkilde. "Intensive Video Gaming Improves Encoding Speed to Visual Short-Term Memory in Young Male Adults." *Acta Psychologica* 142, no. 1 (January 2013): 108–118. DOI: 10.1016/j.actpsy.2012.11.003.

Worley, Susan L. "The Extraordinary Importance of Sleep: The Detrimental Effects of Inadequate Sleep on Health and Public Safety Drive an Explosion of Sleep Research." *Pharmacy and Therapeutics* 43, no. 12 (December 2018): 758–763. PMID: 30559589, PMCID: PMC6281147.

Wu, Aiguo, Zhe Ying, Fernando Gomez-Pinilla. "The Interplay Between Oxidative Stress and Brain-Derived Neurotrophic Factor Modulates the Outcome of a Saturated Fat Diet on Synaptic Plasticity and Cognition." *The European Journal Neuroscience* 19, no 7. (2014): 1699–1707. https://doi.org/10.1111/j.1460-9568.2004.03246.x.

Yaribeygi, Habib, Yunes Panahi, Hedayat Sahraei, Thomas P. Johnston, and Amirhossein Sahebkar. "The Impact of Stress on Body Function: A Review." *EXCLI Journal* 16 (2017): 1057–1072. https://doi.org/10.17179/excli2017–480. PMCID: PMC5579396 PMID: 28900385

Yonelinas, Andrew P., Leun J. Otten, Kendra N. Shaw and Michael D. Rugg. "Separating the Brain Regions Involved in Recollection and Familiarity in Recognition Memory." *Journal of Neuroscience* 25, no. 11 (March 2005): 3002–3008. https://doi.org/10.1523/JNEUROSCI.5295-04.2005.

Yoo, Jeeun, Hongyeop Oh, Seungyeop Jeong, In-Ki Jin. "Comparison of Speech Rate and Long-Term Average Speech Spectrum between Korean Clear Speech and Conversational Speech." *Journal of Audiology & Otology*, 23, no. 4 (October 2019): 187–192. DOI: 10.7874/jao.2019.00115, PMCID: PMC6773961, PMID: 31319638.

Zhan, Lexia, Dingrong Guo, Gang Chen, and Jiongjiong Yang. "Effects of Repetition Learning on Associative Recognition Over Time: Role of the Hippocampus and Prefrontal Cortex." *Frontiers in Human Neuroscience* 12 (July 11, 2018). https://doi.org/10.7874/jao.2019.00115, PMID: 30050418, PMCID: PMC6050388.

Zhang, Jianfen, Na Zhang, Songming Du, Hairong He, Yifan Xu, Hao Cai, Xiaohui Guo, and Guansheng Ma. "The Effects of Hydration Status on Cognitive Performances Among Young Adults in Hebei, China: A Randomized Controlled Trial (RCT)." *International Journal of Environmental Research and Public Health* 15, no. 7 (July 2018): 1477. https://doi.org/10.3390/ijerph15071477, PMCID: PMC6068860 PMID: 30720789.

Zhang, Mingming, Jingwei Zhao, Xiao Li, Xinwang Chen, Jin Xie, Lingyan Meng, and Xiyan Gao. "Effectiveness and Safety of Acupuncture for Insomnia: Protocol for a Systematic Review." *Medicine* 98, no. 45 (2019): e17842. https://doi.org/10.1097/MD.0000000000017842. PMID: 31702639; PMCID: PMC6855569.

Index

adaptation, 144–145
aerobic exercise, *see* exercise
ALS (Lou Gehrig's
    Disease), 181
Alzheimer's, 10, 177, 179, 181,
    183, 185; amyloid-beta
    protein, build-up of, 150
anosognosia, 183
Anti-Mass, 91
Antioxidant foods, 172
associations, the power of,
    142–143
attitudes needing adjustment:
    always right or usually right,
    137, 138–139; going beyond
    thresholds, 137, 139, 142;
    motivation is sufficient,
    137, 146–147; senior
    moments as isolated events,
    137, 142–143; the best,
    accepting only, 137, 143–
    144; unreasonable goals,
    choosing 137, 144–146, 189
automaticity: hippocampus,
    127; making behaviors
    automatic, 128–130;
    removing support, 131;
    testing, 131–133

bad actors: data overload,
    23–24; physiological, 23;
    psychological, 22–23
*Bending Toward Justice:
    The Birmingham Church
    Bombing that Changed the
    Course of Civil Rights*, 91
benzodiazepines, *see* sleep
    medications
Berlin, Isaiah, 65
Bowman, Bob, 127
brain: comparisons, 16,
    97; composition of, 1;
    act-checking, 17, 138;
    functioning, 68, 97–98,
    100; need to sleep,
    156; neurogenesis, 76;
    neurons, 1; plasticity, 79;
    synaptogenesis, 76; weight
    of, 1
The Buddha, 114
Buddhist stories, 4, 111, 114,
    130, 194, 182–183

cannabis, *see* drugs, herbal, supplements, cannabis

Carlin, George, 89

Carter, Jimmy, 184

causation, principle of, 15–16

CBD (cannabidiol), *see* drugs, herbal, supplements, cannabis

CBN (cannabinol) *see* drugs, herbal, supplements, cannabis

change: destination in tiny steps, 56–57; easy, 54–55; experiencing tiny successes, 57–59; rewarding, 60–63; small goals, 55–56

clutter, reducing, 112

Coelho, Paulo, 97

communicative disorders, vii

completing tasks, difficult, 11–12

computer: comparing to the brain, 16; fact-check, 17; features,16, 23; RAM, 23

cognitive creative activities: "what if" scenarios, creating 87–88; activities with constant changes, 81; add something new, 81; beginning new activities, 81; creative writing, 83–84; discussions, participate in, 85–86; existing activities, modify, 80; games, non-electronic, 85; games, video 84–85; getting lost, purposefully 86–87; music, listening differently, 82; puzzles, 82–83

cognitive dissonance, 138–139

cost-benefit analysis, 184

CPAP machines, *see*, sleep devices

creativity, requirements of, 76–77

Curry, Stef, 72

The Dalai Lama, 15

data, reducing speed, *see* noise: data

data, reducing volume, see noise: data

DeGrasse, Neil Tyson, 75

dementia: memory loss, 94, 183; questions about, 187; ruling out, 180–185; seeking help, 177, 182-183, 184–185; statistics, 183–184; structure loss, 13

dependent origination, 15–16

disability, cognition, 56–57, 59

Disney, Walt, 1

disorientation, 13

distractibility, 97–98

doing: add time to complete the activity, 51; reduce the speed, 50–51 drowsiness, *see* fatigue, planning for

drugs: herbal, supplements, cannabis, 163; non-prescription, 163; prescription, 161–162; when to use them, 154–155

dual orexin receptor antagonists, *see* sleep medications

Einstein, Albert, 114

electroencephalogram (EEG), 150

Ellis, Albert, 137

emotions, lessening, 69–70

environment, managing: clutter, reduce, 112–113; internal rules, make external, 108–109; simplify, 114–115; stable settings, replicate, 111; stations, create, 109–111; structure, create, 108; thinking, linearly, 113–114; variables, reduce interfering, 115–116

Erikson, Erik, 7

exercise, 102–103

failures, diagnostic value of, 190–191

fat, saturated, 172

figure-ground, 115, 117–118

fluid intake, *see* hydration

forgetting names and numbers, 9, 58

Franklin, Benjamin, 35

goals: unreasonable, choosing, 144–145

good writing, 45–48

Goodwin, Bryan, 77–86

Gorges, Eric, 78

Gupta, Sanjay, 168

herbal remedies, *see* drugs, herbal, supplements, cannabis

hippocampus, 127

Horowitz, Vladimir, 129

hospice, 116

Huffington, Arianna, 151, 162

hydration, 23, 168–169

identity, 7–8

implants, *see*, sleep devices

inertia, combating, 53–63

information processing: attention, impaired, 16–18; misunderstanding, 18–19; retrieval, inaccurate, 19–21; storage, incomplete or inaccurate, 19; usage, inappropriate, 21–22

Jiyu-Kennett, Abbess, 4

Jones, Doug, 91

Kabat-Zinn, Jon, 100
Kau, Michio, 15

language learning: adult, 81;
    child, 20
Larson, Doug, 167
listening: framework, create
    written, 40–41; simulation,
    interaction, 41–42; slow
    down, asking speaker
    to, 37–39; speed bump,
    introduce, 39–40

macro-nutrients, *see* nutrition
magnetic resonance imaging
    (MRI), 20
Maraboli, Steve, 107
melatonin receptor antagonists,
    see sleep medications
metabolic homeostasis, *see*
    nutrition
micro-nutrients, *see also*
    nutrition
Miller, Kirsten, 77–86
memory: conflating, 12;
    creating, 90–93; direct
    evidence, 27; episodic,
    82–83; feature-poor, 90;
    feature-rich, 89–90, 91–92;
    hooks, retrieval, 90, 190;
    injury-based guesses,
    27–28; intervention-based
    guesses, 28; long-term,
    28, 30; observation-based

guesses, 27; retrieving,
    93–96; sensory (iconic)
    memory, 28, 29; sequential,
    29, 30; short-term memory,
    28, 29, 53–54; storage, 19;
    three-dimensional pictures,
    26; trace, 142; types
    8- 13; working (executive
    function) memory, 29, 30,
    187
memory aides: connections,
    creating, 92; multisensory,
    91–92; repetitive
    vocalizations, 92–93
methods, definition of, 33
Miller, Kirsten, 77–86
mindfulness, 34: definition,
    99–100; prioritizing,
    34, 101–102; switching
    activities, 103; taking breaks,
    102–103
monitoring: physical behaviors,
    99; speech acts, 98
motivation, 60–61, 146–147
music, how to listen, 82
myths, 4; grouped together, 4,
    5; inevitable part of aging,
    4, 6; isolated events, 4, 7;
    laughable, 4, 7; momentary
    brain glitches, 4, 5; result
    only of memory problems,
    4, 6

naps, *see* fatigue, planning for

National Institute of Health (NIH), 183
Newton, Isaac, 53
noise: data, 119–121; external, 21, 97, 115, 116–118; internal, 21, 97, 118–119
noise maskers, *see*, sleep devices
nutrition: carbohydrates, high-glycemic-load, 173; curcumin, 170; flavonoids, 170; folate or folic acid, 171; foods, fried, 173; nitrates, 173–174; omega-3 fatty acids, 170; sugar, added, 172

objects, misplacing, 10

Parker, Cornelia, 91
patterns: disrupting old, 67; erecting a wall to stop the progression, 70; finding them, 189; lessening emotions, 69–70; memorization, 73–74; repetition, 72–73; triggers, creating, 71; triggers, eliminating, 68–69
perception, 83
Phelps, Mark, 127
phenomenology, 100–101
physics, first law, 53
Popeye, 7–8, 195

practice: consistency, 111, 130; how, 127–128; identifying salient features, 128; intention, need for, 72–73; repetition, 129–130; structure, 124–128; what, 126–127; when, 125–126; where, 124–125
processing skills, 187
procrastination, 12, 90
punishment, 60

questions, frequently asked, 187–191

reading: contents, subdivide, 45–46; format, change, 49; quiet, 48–49; reading rate, reduce, 43- 44; scanning, 44; units, beginning and end, 47–48
reinforcement: extraneous, 62; extrinsic, 62; intrinsic, 61
retrieval aides: cues and tags, 93–94; lists, 95; numbers, 95–96
Ronald Reagan, 184
rules, making internal external, 108–109
Rumsfeld, Donald, 175, 180

Sagan, Carl, 163
senior moments: common approaches, 3; completing

tasks, 11–12; conflating memories, 12; context, 17–18; definition of, 3; disorientation, 13; forgetting, 9; misplacing objects, 10; myths, 3–8; repeating, 9–10; return, 190; sequencing, 11; significance, 179–180; types, 8- 13; understanding, 12–13

seniors counselor, vii

sequencing problems, 11

Shakespeare, William, 149

simplifying, 114–115

Skinner, B.F., 27; black box, 27, 68

sleep, 23; alcohol drinking, when to stop, 156–157; circadian rhythm, 153; cognitive behavior therapy (CBT), 152; darkness, 153; deprivation, 156; eating, when to stop, 155–156; exercise, 164–165; fatigue, planning for, 165; lack of, 21; light-emitting diodes (LEDs), 158; medications, 161–163; meditation, 34, 158–159, 105–106; noise, 153; REM sleep, 150, 152, 154; sleep devices, 159–161; sleep environment, creating a, 152–153; temperature, 152–153; timing

interventions for maximum effect, 154–158

The Sleep Revolution, 151, 162

slowing down: doing, 49–51; listening, 36–42; reading, 43–49; troubleshooting, 188

Stanford Sleep Medicine Center, 150, 151

Stay Sharp: Build a Better Brain at Any Age

strategies: challenge the brain, 75–88; combating inertia, 53–63; compensating for aging, 6; definition, 33; focus, 97–106, 107; fortifying and retrieving memories 89–96; managing your environment, 107–121; methods, 33–34; modifying, 177–178, 188; patterns, 65–74; practice, 123–133; slow down, 35–51; troubleshooting, 178–179, 188

stress, reducing, 103; choosing appropriate goals, 104, 146; completing tasks, 104–105; meditating, 105–106

structure: creating, 108; loss of, 13

substituting words, 10

supplements, *see* drugs, herbal, supplements, cannabis

systematic desensitization, 69

Talfel, Henri, 7

THC (tetrahydrocannabionol) *see also* drugs, herbal, supplements, cannabis

thinking: linear, 113–114; multitasking, avoiding, 21, 113, 114

thresholds: cognitive, 141–142; exceeding, 139–140; physical, 140–141

Tutu, Desmond Bishop, 53, 55

understanding, difficulty, 12

visual scanning, 83

visualization, 34

vitamins, b, c, d, e, 171

weighted blankets, *see*, sleep devices

Welch, Jack, 33

xenophobia, 38

Z sedative-hypnotics, *see* sleep medications

About the Author

Stan Goldberg, PhD, professor emeritus at San Francisco State University, has written 195 articles, seven chapters, and nine books published in four languages. He has received 26 national and international awards including Best Buddhist Writings of 2010 (along with Thich Nhat Hanh) and The London Book Festival Grand Prize Winner. His website is stangoldbergwriter.com.

Printed in the USA
CPSIA information can be obtained
at www.ICGtesting.com
LVHW090900161023
759509LV00030B/9